Instead of Watching TV

99 Activities to Help Kids Unplug

Anna Huete

Translated by Julie Ganz

D1456908

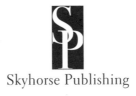

Skyhorse Publishing

Original title: EN VEZ DE VER LA TELE
© 2005 by Editorial Océano, S.L. (Barcelona, Spain)

English translation © 2015 by Skyhorse Publishing

Skyhorse Publishing books may be purchased in bulk at special
discounts for sales promotion, corporate gifts, fund-raising, or
educational purposes. Special editions can also be created to
specifications. For details, contact the Special Sales Depart-
ment, Skyhorse Publishing, 307 West 36th Street, 11th Floor,
New York, NY 10018 or info@skyhorsepublishing.com.

Skyhorse® and Skyhorse Publishing® are registered trademarks
of Skyhorse Publishing, Inc.®, a Delaware corporation.

Visit our website at www.skyhorsepublishing.com.

10 9 8 7 6 5 4 3 2 1

Library of Congress Cataloging-in-Publication Data is available
on file.

Cover design by Qualcom Design
Cover photo credit: Thinkstock

ISBN: 978-1-62914-470-2
Ebook ISBN: 978-1-63220-007-5
Printed in China

Contents

Introduction

It is Sunday morning, the week has been very hard, but my small "monster" has decided that today he wants to get up early. Thus, at eight o'clock I have already eaten breakfast and started to give in to the clear evidence that it is more useful to do some work around the house while my child entertains himself with some of his toys. But the break does not last long, and though I intend to clean up the kitchen and to start the washing machine, my child starts to wander around without knowing what to do, touching everything and disorganizing everything I had just cleaned. He is bored and asks me if he can watch TV. But my principles as a mom, who wants the best for her child, don't allow it and I encourage him to play with the endless list of toys that he has in his room. Nevertheless, my little one doesn't comply and starts to rebel. It is very early and the temptation, as on other occasions, is great. I know that with only the press of a button, he will be still and silent for quite some time, and I will be able to enjoy a relaxed Sunday morning. He also knows that I know it, and thus he does not stop insisting. The TV, on this occasion, would serve as the perfect babysitter.

Surely this picture is familiar to you and we don't need to tell the rest of the story, right? But how would it seem if we change the story, so that instead, the child finds other ways of entertaining himself without having to resort to the television?

In the following pages we propose up to ninety-nine fun and didactic alternatives that will allow you to enjoy a good time in the company of your child, and will even allow your young one to discover the great pleasure of entertaining himself/herself.

It is worth it, don't you think?

Recent studies reveal that children in Spain spend more than three hours daily (218 minutes) in front of the TV. Although this medium of communication is a screen that is available to the world and provides many good things, there is no doubt that it is the job of the parents to control kids' consumption of television and, most of all, to promote its rational use. Diverse studies have shown that kids should spend only thirty minutes a day in front of the TV. If they surpass this time, it increases the risk of obesity and small behavioral issues. Don't forget either that it is necessary to sit at least 5 feet (1.5 m) from the apparatus to avoid vision problems.

Watching TV is a passive activity. The child is sitting still, almost mute, in front of a huge source of visual stimulants. He/she doesn't run, he/she doesn't move, and he/she doesn't interact with other children, something that is essential during the first years of his/her life.

And, in addition, TV is not the only temptation. In recent decades items known as "new screens" have appeared, such as the computer and video games. These products have changed the play and leisure habits of our children, and also those of some adults. One of the first clear consequences that this new form of entertainment has produced is the alarming increase of child obesity, but it has other less visible, though equally undesirable, effects as well, such as lack of communication between kids and between parents and children, decrease in the use of their imagination, or difficulties concentrating. The result is a passive, solitary, and less creative child, who spends hours and hours in front of a computer or TV.

Although it may not seem like it to you, your own house can be a tireless source of leisurely resources to share. It is our obligation as parents to cultivate in our children an interest in discovering things to do at home that are a true alternative to watching television. It all helps to prevent turning to the TV out of laziness, out of inertia, or for the comfort of the parent. We, as parents, often promote its excessive use as the only object of entertainment.

Without a doubt, you don't have an excuse anymore. We offer you ninety-nine entertaining activities that are so fun that you will not remember to turn on the television and, more importantly, neither will your kids. If your kids are between four and ten years old they will find, via these kinds of activities, their primary source of growth and diversion. Take note, and have fun watching how they enjoy, grow, and learn!

How to watch TV

Inevitably, watching TV has become habitual and impressionable in the majority of homes. Kids are used to it from a very early age and, at times, they spend too many hours in front of it. Can it damage them to watch it when they are young? Teachers and psychologists worldwide have contemplated this question and the response has been almost unanimous: TV in and of itself is not good or bad; it all depends on its use.

Although it may seem that TV is a threat to the education of our children, in reality it is the indiscriminate, unlimited use that has become of it that is the threat. To watch TV is one of the most important and most influential pastimes in the lives of kids and adolescents. And, while it can entertain, inform, and accompany kids, it can also influence them in an undesirable way. From four to five years of age, kids establish permanent habits and emotional characteristics, through imitation and identification. Imitation is conscious, but identification is unconscious and occurs from the adoption of standards of conduct and attitudes of those who are important to them.

For that reason, it is necessary to be attentive to the effects that TV can have on the child, above all in reference to violent content. Violent scenes can generate aggressive conduct in children, via the simple means of learning and imitating them. If the parents agree that the kids can watch TV, first they should be sure that they have positive experiences with the TV.

On the other hand, the time that a child spends in front of the TV takes away from other important activities such as reading, schoolwork, playtime, interaction with family, and social development. In addition, through the television, kids can learn things that are not appropriate or correct, yet many times they don't know the difference between the fantasy that is presented to them and reality. They are under the influence of the thousands of public announcements that they see every year, many of which are for alcoholic beverages, unhealthy foods, fast food, and toys. On the other hand, the exaggerated representation of "perfect" body images can contribute to the problem of anorexia, above all in adolescents, due to the anxiety that it provokes. If an overweight child learns from the TV the importance of staying in shape, in an exaggerated way, he or she is going to develop complexes and consequently will follow the advice and the diets that the TV projects, aside from the erroneous values that he/she will be assimilating.

And as if all that weren't enough, the television also exposes kids to types of behaviors and attitudes that are difficult to understand, like violence, sexuality, race and gender stereotypes, and drug and alcohol abuse. Impressionable kids and adolescents can assume that that which they see on TV is normal, and that it is safe and acceptable.

Finally, the facts show that kids who watch too much TV have greater risk of getting bad grades, reading less, doing less exercise, and talking less with the other members of the family. There are too many "negative" effects not to notice them. Without a doubt, watching TV with your kids can result in a beneficial experience for everyone, although it may not seem it for all of the aforementioned reasons. In the programming of all the TV channels, there exists space dedicated to the young crowd—documentaries, films, and craft programs that are very entertaining, and that awaken the imagination and a sense of creativity. You, the parents, can help your kids have positive experiences with the television by watching those programs with your kids. Without a doubt, it is advisable that you choose the most appropriate ones for the development level of your young one, that you put time limits on TV watching for your kids, that you don't watch it during eating or studying times, and that you don't permit them to watch the programs that seem inappropriate for them.

In addition to preventing kids from watching TV for consecutive hours, you can also stimulate discussions with them about what you are watching when you watch a show together, pointing out positive behaviors like cooperation, friendship, and taking an interest in others. Another possibility that watching TV together offers you is to make connections with history, books, places of interest, and personal events, by talking to them about personal and familial values and how they relate to what they are watching in the program, or asking the kids to compare the contents with real-life events.

You could also teach them to have a critical vision about what you are watching by educating them on the true consequences of violence from images of particular movies. Or you can also discuss with them the role of publicity and its influence on what you buy.

As you can see, with the appropriate orientation, the child can learn to use the television in a healthy, positive way, and to take advantage of an omnipresent medium in all homes. Without a doubt, you should never forget to stimulate your children so pastimes, sports, and friends of their age surround them. The ideal solution resides, as always, in a good balance.

How to prevent addiction to television

- **Encourage active recreation.** Get your child interested in sports, games, crafts, and music. From time to time, turn off the TV and go for a walk or play with your child.

- **Read to your kids.** Start to read to your kids from when they are a year old and encourage them to read by themselves when they grow older. Some parents allow for TV or video game time to be equivalent to the time the child spends reading. Help them improve their aptitudes for conversing by spending more time talking with them.

- **Limit the time spent watching TV to two hours a day or fewer.** An alternative is to limit TV to an hour on school nights and to two or three hours a day on weekends. You can permit them more time when there is a special educational program on.

- **It is not a distraction.** Don't use TV as a distraction or as a babysitter for preschool-aged children. TV for these kids should be limited to special programs produced for small children. As the difference between fantasy and reality at this age isn't clear, normal programs can provoke fears.

- **Duties first.** If the child is doing badly in school, limit the TV time to a half hour a day. Establish a rule so that the child should finish his/her household duties and obligations first before watching TV. If his/her favorite program is on before finishing his/her homework, you can tape it so he/she can watch it later.

- **Go to sleep on time.** Establish bedtime without altering it for a program that can interest your child. Kids who are allowed to stay up late watching TV normally are very tired the next day when they need to be attentive and receptive to what is being taught in school. Don't permit your child to have a TV in the room, because this limits the control that you have over the time that he/she is watching it.

- **Turn off the TV during meals.** Family time is too valuable to blow it on TV programs. In addition, don't always use the TV as background music in your house. If you don't like a silent house, plan to listen to music without a melody.

- **Teach him/her to choose the programs with good judgment.** Turn on the TV only to watch specific programs. Don't leave it to chance to look for an interesting program afterward. Teach your child to consult the program guide before turning on the TV.

- **Teach him/her to turn off the TV when a program ends.** If the TV stays on, your child probably will be interested in the following program and then it will become more difficult to leave the TV.

- **Stimulate your child so that he/she watches educational programs** or those that teach human values. Stimulate him/her so that he/she watches documentaries or real-life dramas. Use the programs about love, sex, family disputes, alcoholism, and drugs as a form of initiating family discussions about difficult topics.

- **Prohibit violent programs.** This signifies that you should know what your child is watching and should turn off the TV if the program he/she is watching doesn't seem appropriate. This can also include the daily news.

  Make lists separated by the programs that are appropriate for both small and big kids to watch. Make the older kids more responsible for making sure the younger ones are outside of the room where the TV is when they watch programs not permitted for the younger kids. If they don't comply, the channel should be changed.

  If you allow your child to watch programs that contain violence, speak to him/her about the consequences of doing so.

  Tell them about the form in which violence damages the victim and the victim's family. If your child is bothered by a program that he/she has seen, assure him/her by talking about it.

- **Discuss the news with your children.** Help them identify those commercials with a high degree of pressure to sell and that make exaggerated claims. If your child wants a toy based on a TV personality, ask him/her how he/she is going to use it in the house. The response will probably convince you that the toy will serve to grow the collection more than convert it into a catalyst of active play.

- **Explain the differences between fantasy and reality.** This type of clarification can help your child enjoy a program and, without a doubt, understand that what is happening on TV could not happen in real life.

- **Set an example.** If you spend a lot of time watching TV, you can be sure that your child will do the same. In addition, the types of programs that you watch send a very clear message to your child.

Playing is so much fun

It is possible that your experience until today makes you believe that your young ones don't like anything else besides TV and video games. But your kids, like all kids, like to play, and in addition they need to do so to have other experiences that help them learn and develop intellectually.

And when we talk to you about playing, we are not referring to expensive toys or amusement parks, but rather to helping them explore their surroundings and accompanying them on that expedition while you dedicate yourself to the work you have to do each day. Kids can have fun sharing very simple things with their parents.

Although it can seem like an exaggeration, almost whatever object that you're surrounded with in your house or at the park can be used to play with. In actuality, all toys come assembled and packed, ready for consumption. But it is much more fun, and creative, to find toys where it seems unlikely or to make them with your own hands. Thus, we learn that the creation of toys forms part of a fun moment that you can share with your kids.

For example, making a ball. We already know that there are very few children who can resist playing when a ball is present. But it can still be very fun to encourage them to look for paper or cloths around the house, to give shape to them, and to tie them with an adhesive seal. With this they make a ball that is not too hard to be able to play with inside the house and they will have spent a good time making it. You will have figured out that the time dedicated to the game increases and also becomes a creative moment.

Another example that can help is that of cardboard boxes. How many times have you found yourself surprised that your child plays more with the box that contains his birthday toy than with the toy itself?! And boxes open a whole world of possibilities, from an improvised sled to a dollhouse or a theater. And if the box is from the refrigerator that you just bought, there are endless possibilities and the games that it inspires could occupy many subsequent afternoons.

And another great ally of good times is the imagination. There is nothing as rich and as missed on some occasions. To shoot and pass an imaginary ball, for example, will help you exercise the musculature and have you laughing from satisfaction. All, simply, thanks to your imagination.

In the pages that follow you will find crafts, games to practice inside the house, simple cooking recipes, and exciting science experiments so your kids and their friends remain surprised each time. There are easy challenges that open ninety-nine different possibilities to you, rather than watching TV. So what are you waiting for?

Our work as parents requires dedication and sacrifice, but should not always be an arduous, difficult commitment. The idleness of our children is an ideal means to being able to teach them values such as generosity, honesty, or respect for others, not to mention its ability to increase their manual abilities and creativity.

In this fun educational facet emerge board games (which are of great help), to which we have dedicated so many hours in our infancy. We are referring to Parcheesi, cards, the goose game, playing with boats, checkers, or chess. You can teach them how you played and share with them a good time.

The kitchen also offers you the possibility of entertaining your kids in a very tasty way. With your help they will be able to make simple recipes and discover the pleasure of giving their loved ones, and themselves, delicious dishes and sweet desserts.

Very simple crafts

Walnut turtles

Walnuts are delicious and very nutritious, but they can also be recycled and converted into a funny turtle. The steps are very simple and your child will spend some very enjoyable moments with them.

- **Age:** 6–10 years
- **Number of participants:** as few as one
- **Space:** wherever
- **Materials:**
    *pastel colors
    *shells of different kinds of nuts
    *short needle pins (for walls)
- **Method:** Help your child split the nut in two, so that the shells are symmetrical and perfect. Afterward, the shell should be empty, to be filled completely with a pastel. With it, you will have obtained the body of this popular turtle and the base from which you can work to create these funny turtles.

Next, and with the same pastel color with which you made the tummy of the animal, make the feet and head with different nuts, four small and one large. Afterward, with a different color make two small balls for the eyes and a small cylinder for the mouth. The child can also get the effect of the eyes with the short-cut pins. At the head he/she should mold the neck, with which the shell will be united. In addition, the child should also make the tail. Once he/she has all the parts that project from the shell of the turtle, the only thing left is to stick them to one another. And that's it. I hope you don't throw away the shells of the other nuts. You can make a whole family of turtles, or create snails and dinosaurs, with them.

The blind drawing

All kids like to draw, that is clear. But what seems difficult is to add to the act of drawing an incentive so that it becomes a game. That is solely what we are proposing in this blind drawing activity.

- **Age:** 6–10 years
- **Number of participants:** at least one
- **Space:** wherever
- **Materials:**
    * pencil
    * paper, better when it's a big size
    * handkerchief to cover the eyes
- **Method:** Ask your child to sit at a desk or table. Show him/her the paper on which to draw and the pencil or marker that he/she is going to use. Agree with him/her before starting on which object or animal he/she wants to draw and, next, blindfold his/her eyes with a handkerchief.

The child should plan to draw the best possible animal or object that you have agreed upon and afterward can laugh at the result.

Variable: More players can participate. Then, agree to say into someone's ear the animal that you will draw, and afterward show all the drawings to the participants so that they can guess what you had wanted to draw in each case.

Strange characters

Cutting and pasting is a fun activity that you can do your whole life, but to recreate characters by combining various elements of different beings, animals, or things is a challenge that kids don't usually resist. As soon as you propose the idea, they will put their hands to the task.

- **Age:** 5–10 years
- **Number of participants:** at least one
- **Space:** wherever
- **Materials:**
    * old magazines
    * colors
    * paper or cardboard
    * round-pointed scissors
    * glue
    * colored yarn
    * cotton
- **Method:** Although kids love to clip animals and characters from magazines, there are activities that can still boost the pleasure of snipping the back pages from the tabloids or the newspaper.
    The idea is to create strange characters by combining different people or animals. For example, you can paint on a paper a dinosaur and

put the head of a famous movie actor on top, or cut out the figure of an esteemed actress and add to it the feet of an astronaut and the head of a bearded governor. In addition, you can personalize the result, sticking strands of yarn to put long hair on a distinguished bald man or a cotton beard on the front of a horse.

In whichever combination, the results are usually funny and the kids don't usually come up with just one "creation," which enables them to have a good time while they prepare it and when they discuss it with you or with their father upon his arrival home from work.

Calendar

Each Christmas, many calendars that we don't usually use arrive at the house. With a little imagination, your child can personalize one so that it serves as a guide to familiar events, such as sacred holidays, birthdays, and wedding anniversaries. It can also help in planning school trips or extracurricular activities.

- **Age:** 7–11 years
- **Number of participants:** at least one
- **Space:** wherever
- **Materials:**
    * a gridded calendar
    * colored markers
    * white labels
- **Method:** To make this craft, you need a calendar with a slightly large grid that fits the labels. Once chosen, ask your child to draw on the labels as many birthday desserts as there are members of your family. He/she should do the same with all of the events that you wish to mark: a backpack or a bus for excursions, a gift for sacred days, a beach ball or umbrella for summer vacations, a Santa head for Christmas . . . When he/she has made the labels, help him/her

go through the months of the upcoming year and indicate on which days he/she should stick the labels. If you have permanent markers you can draw directly on the calendar. Ask him/her to also write the name of the honoree to best identify the anniversary or birthday. Each page that you arrange while you pass through the year will be a symbol of that fun winter afternoon that the two of you spent personalizing the calendar.

Newspaper drawings

With this craft, kids are entertained using materials that they don't generally use to create drawings or murals. Thus they learn to observe their environment in order to find creative materials and they learn to recycle.

- **Age:** 8–10 years
- **Number of participants:** at least one
- **Space:** wherever
- **Materials:**
    * dark-colored poster board
    * newspaper
    * pencil
    * round-pointed scissors
    * glue
- **Method:** In this craft, you get surprising results from something that upon first glance doesn't seem artistic—the newspaper. Your child should think about easy silhouettes to cut out, such as mountains, houses, planes, clouds, etc., and draw them with a pencil on the newspaper. Next, cut these out and place them on the dark poster board. Afterward, glue them, and thus you will have obtained a surprising combination with simple materials that are always around the house.

House with windows

Kids love to paint, glue, cut . . . They can spend whole hours doing so. But, at times, they are done with their ideas and they let out the feared phrase of "I am bored." The idea that we propose next satisfies that pleasure for crafts but with a different, very pleasing result. Certainly, your child will be very content after having created his/her house with windows like the real ones.

- **Age:** 7–11 years
- **Number of participants:** at least one
- **Space:** wherever
- **Materials:**
  - * piercing tool
  - * poster board
  - * pencil
  - * clear blue cellophane
  - * round-pointed scissors
  - * glue
  - * markers or colored pencils
  - * ruler
- **Method:** Your child will be able to create a house with windows and a door that opens. It is very easy. He/she should draw the façade of the house on the poster board and, with the help of something that can be used for piercing, such as a filed pencil, retrace the lines of the windows and the entrance door, jabbing it to make holes that are close together. At the end, the board will break on the dotted line (it can be helped using scissors) and it will enable them to open the windows and door. To get a cleaner bend, ask that he/she place the ruler on the hinge line and that he/she then double the pages of the windows and the entrance door.

Once this is done, he/she can make a new "cutting line" inside the windows. When he/she has "emptied" the glass pane, he/she can glue to the outside part a square of the clear blue (or whatever color he/she prefers) cellophane, for the middle of the window. With that, he/she will have the effect of a crystal window and will be able to see through it.

Next he/she can draw on another poster board the silhouette of the façade and create the corresponding rooms with furniture. Afterward, he/she can glue the façade by the borders and thus the rooms will be seen through the closed windows.

This technique can also be applied to postcards and other crafts that require transparencies.

Fun monster

We propose a craft that takes advantage of the egg cartons that we always throw out and that can be converted into fun monsters with big mouths. At the very least, they are always a good excuse to spend a fun time and to increase your child's creativity.

- **Age:** 6–10 years
- **Number of participants:** at least one
- **Space:** wherever
- **Materials:**
    * a half-dozen egg carton
    * brush
    * colored paint
    * colored wool
    * glue
- **Method:** After covering the area in which your child is going to work with old newspaper, tell him/her to start painting the inside

and outside of the carton in its entire-ty, with the color that he/she likes. When it has dried, he/she should paint a white eye with a black pupil (or whichever color he/she prefers) on each side where the carton is opened. He/she can make it very expressive with the help of eye-brows, eyelashes, or whatever occurs to him/her, from a star-shaped eye to a double eye on each side. To make this monster's hair, there is a very simple method. Make a mane of wool attached to the center and cut around on each side. In this way, there will be a clump in the middle and a mountain of uncombed "hairs" on each side. When it has this wig, it should be glued to the top part, above the eyes, and we will have just made this fun monster. The mouth is the box itself that opens and closes, and it can trap more than a curious hand that wants to mess up its hair. If you want you can paint the edges in red and some teeth on the lower part. The limit exists only in your imagination, as always.

Create a kite

A kite is a toy from more than three thousand years ago. Since then, it has been present in children's games, although the lack of open spaces and time to ded-icate to the free air has reduced its presence at beaches on summer afternoons. Without a doubt, it is a fun activity, and here we teach you to make it with your own hands.

- **Age:** at least five years old
- **Number of participants:** at least one

- **Space:** in the house and in free air
- **Materials:**
  - * a plastic bag
  - * 2 fine sticks of wood, bamboo, or metal
  - * string
  - * strong adhesive tape
  - * cord for kites
  - * a reel or handle
  - * acrylic paint
  - * a brush
- **Method:** The process is simple, although a little laborious, and so you should help your child follow these steps:

  From the plastic bag, cut a square-like shape, with two sides longer than the other two. Cut sticks of the same size as the kite. Cross the sticks and attach them in the center. With that, it becomes the base, or, that is to say, the structure of the kite.

  With the structure done, glue it with adhesive tape on the kite. Turn it over and put a piece of adhesive tape on the cross of the structure. In this way, the plastic will be protected when you pass the cord. Immediately, cut a piece of cord for kites, double the size of the kite's height. Sew or pass a side of the cord through the front part of the kite and roll the center of the structure various times and return it to the front. Attach rigidly. This is the flange.

  Turn the kite around. Pass the other side of the cord through the lower part of the kite and stretch with caution until it is rigid. Attach the flight cord to the flange, a little above the center, adjusting it when you try the kite.

  Now decorate the kite. You can use soapy water so that the paint dries up better on the plastic. Then make the tail. The tail is what gives the kite stability. Make one with plastic, five times the height of the kite.

Now you just have to find a free moment of the day with wind to get to a big park, the beach, or whatever free space you find nearby to test your fantastic kite.

Caution: Before making a kite, it is very important to talk to your child about how and where you will fly it afterward. It is necessary to consider some basic rules:

- You should never fly a kite close to electricity lines and poles.
- Metal cords or materials should **not** be used on the kite. That would attract electricity.
- It is advisable to use fishing wire or special wire for kites.
- Don't use the kite when it is raining. Wet cords could attract electricity.
- In the case that the kite is stuck in a tree or post, it is best to leave it there and not try to capture it. Climbing to high-up places is dangerous.
- The kite should be flown in places where there is no one nearby. An uncontrolled fall by your kite could bother other people.
- The kite should not be flown near highways; it can distract drivers.
- Nor should you use the kite when the conditions are stormy.

Mr. Lawn

This activity will serve as an excuse to explain to your child how a plant grows. It is composed of various phases. In the first, it becomes a zygote in a nice pot. Afterward, wait a few days while the seeds, which your child will have excitedly planted, grow, and, finally, after a week he/she will have a plant to take care of and a fun Mr. Lawn to show his/her friends.

- **Age:** at least four years old
- **Number of participants:** at least one
- **Space:** wherever

- **Materials:**
  * eggshells
  * round-pointed scissors
  * cotton
  * canary grass seeds
  * temperas or permanent markers
- **Method:** To be able to make this craft, you should remove the upper part of an egg and empty it.

  When you decide that your child is making the Mr. Lawn craft, tell him/her to cut with caution the edges of the shells with scissors. Afterward, he/she can draw on it, with temperas or permanent markers, eyes, a nose, ears, a mouth, and, if he/she wants, a mustache on Mr. Lawn and bows or a ponytail on Mrs. Plant.

  When he/she has made the "flowerpot stand," he/she should fill it with a little cotton, without totally filling it. On top of the cotton, help him/her put various seeds, which should stay totally covered by the cotton.

  Now all that's left is to pray and to wait a couple of days. Meanwhile, make sure it is in a bright place and that he/she adds a little bit more water every day. In a week, the eggshell with the Mr. Lawn or Mrs. Plant face will have developed a precious green head of hair.

Playing-card costume

There are many ways to make an effective and inexpensive costume that is full of imagination. Here we propose a playing-card costume that is very easy to make and that requires few materials. Surely, your kids will love it as much as their friends will and at the next carnival they will be dressed up as a deck of cards.

- **Age:** 8–12 years

- **Number of participants:** at least one
- **Space:** wherever
- **Materials:**
  - * wrapping paper
  - * round-pointed scissors
  - * wax crayons
  - * brush
  - * gel
- **Method:** You should cut a piece of wrapping paper that measures more or less double the size of your child. Next, double it in the middle and trace a semicircle. Upon cutting it out you will have the hole through which your child will "wear" the costume. You should realize that it has to be sufficiently big so that it fits over the child's head.

  With the wax crayons he/she will be able to paint the motif of the letter that he/she likes most. When it is finished, paint it with gel so that the wrapping paper acquires a brilliant finish and the colors look more alive. And already, the costume is done.

Kaleidoscope

When our children are preadolescents it is most difficult to entertain them with games or crafts, but the kaleidoscope is an instrument that attracts them via the magic of the colors and the geometric shapes that they see. It is pretty certain that they would love the idea of constructing one and understanding its function. So let's get to work!

- **Age:** 9–11 years
- **Number of participants:** at least one
- **Space:** wherever

- **Materials:**
  - cardboard or plastic tube 6.3 inches (16 cm) in length and 2 inches (5 cm) in diameter
  - rectangular mirrors $^8/_{10}$ inch by 6.3 inches (2 cm by 16 cm)
  - adhesive tape
  - cardboard lid that is the diameter of the tube (one, in which you will add a hole through which to look)
  - 3 glass or plastic transparencies, circular, of the same diameter as the tube (of a bottle or of plastic sheets)
  - semitransparent paper (waxed paper or tracing paper)
  - colored paper (to decorate)
  - plastic pieces, beads, or whatever occurs to you
  - round-pointed scissors

  Note: You can get the mirrors and glass circles in a glassware store (they always have leftovers). The plastic circles are made with acetate sheets, bottles, or plastic jars. Tell your child to be cautious with these materials; they shouldn't press them with force or touch them a lot because they can get cut.

- **Method:** First, he/she should take the mirrors and place them one next to the other (leaving a small space in between) and facedown, atop a table. Afterward, tell him/her to place two pieces of adhesive tape on top and to turn over the mirrors.

  Next, he/she should move the mirrors so that they make up a triangle with the mirrored side facedown (like a small triangular box). Afterward, place the triangle of mirrors inside the cardboard tube, surrounding it with newspaper so that it does not move. And put one of the plastic or glass circles on one side of the tube.

  Afterward, he/she should make a small hole in the middle of the cardboard lid and glue it over the glass (so he/she will be able to see what is happening inside of the kaleidoscope). On the other side, he/she should place another glass circle. And, finally, he/she should put a piece of wax paper on top of this circle. As the last artistic touch, he/she can paint the tube with vinyl adhesive and afterward glue colored paper to it.

And already, he/she will have just made a pretty kaleidoscope. Now he/she will be able to look through the hole, pointing the other end toward the light. At the same time that he/she turns the tube, he/she will see distinct geometric shapes of many colors.

Art with crayons

This kind of creation is very simple and original. In addition, it can help you recycle the pieces of crayons that always seem to be around and with which it is not possible to color because they are too small. Although your child will need you for the ironing of the drawing, the rest of the craft can be achieved alone or in the company of their siblings or friends. It is a pretty way to decorate your refrigerator or the cork on the wall of the studio.

- **Age:** whatever
- **Number of participants:** at least one
- **Space:** wherever
- **Materials:**
    * 2 sheets of tracing paper of the same size
    * different color crayons
    * sticky tape
    * an old grater
    * an iron
- **Method:** Tell your child to place one of the papers on top of a flat surface appropriately protected by some old newspapers or an oil-cloth. Next, he/she should take the grater and, cautiously, grate the different color crayons on top of the paper.

Once the colors are grated, ask him/her to distribute them in the way that he/she desires. He/she can do it based on a previous drawing or let his/her imagination fly and create an abstract drawing. When the drawing is done, he/she should put the other piece of paper on top and attach it with some pieces of tape so that the shreds don't move.

At this stage of the craft is when you enter, as you should turn on the iron at a low temperature and, when it is hot, run it on top of the papers so the crayon shreds melt and stick to the two surfaces. The final drawing is a beautiful sketch of colors that blur and that, once cooled, can decorate any wall of your home or workplace.

Scattered comic

From the story created by the original comic artist, your child can dedicate a good time to trimming, gluing, thinking, and reading, while barely realizing that time has passed. You should help him/her only a little and the rest he/she will do on his/her own. If he/she prefers, he/she can always invent his/her own order and create a comic with silly, senseless dialogue and absurd situations.

- **Age:** 5–10 years
- **Number of participants:** however many
- **Space:** wherever
- **Materials:**
  * a comic book
  * round-pointed scissors
  * glue
  * a sheet of notebook drawing paper or that of the mural kind (A3)
- **Method:** Ask your child to choose a comic story that he/she likes and help him/her cut out the cartoons. Next, you should cut out the dialogue bubbles and set them aside.

Once you've cut them out, hand over the dialogue bubbles in a pile so that the child can order them and paste them in the corresponding spots. Once this enjoyable "jigsaw puzzle" is over, ask him/her to read you the final story to figure out if he/she has done the game correctly.

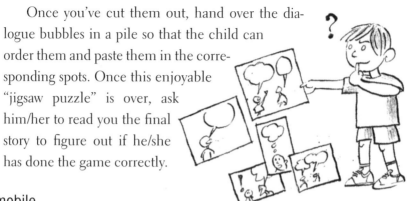

Angel mobile

When our children are babies we hang a mobile toy over their crib to calm them and to help them sleep. When they grow, the attraction that this object has to them is not lost, but rather they still love having it hang from the ceiling of their room and spending a long time looking at it. This mobile project has the ability to also entertain the children while they make it. It's a win-win for you.

- **Age:** 6–10 years
- **Number of participants:** at least one
- **Space:** wherever
- **Materials:**
    * resistant paper
    * color poster board
    * glue
    * round-pointed scissors
    * pencil
    * brush
    * temperas
    * threads
    * 2 pencils or wooden rods
- **Method:** Although the principal motif of this mobile is a bunch of small angels, your child can also choose peacocks, swans, squirrels,

or whatever other motif. When he/she has decided, he/she should take the sheets of paper and fold them like an accordion. It is advisable to mark the folds well, squeezing them with your fingers.

Once the sheets are folded, he/she should double one of their points in a hook shape and glue them. From the other point they will be able to open, like a fan.

Now, ask him/her to draw silhouettes of the angel figures, which are going to serve as a base, on the poster board. To make the figures, he/she should paint the fans with colors and go over the outline of the figures with black.

To construct the mobile, he/she should hang the silhouettes on two rods or pencils forming a cross and fasten them by means of a fishing line or a color cord. And to finish, he/she should fasten the figures at the four extremes of the cross. And now it is ready to hang wherever the child prefers.

Decorated leaves

Autumn converts the streets into carpets of big leaves of beautiful yellow bananas. For our small artists, those leaves provide them with an opportunity to express themselves and create beautiful works of art. With few materials and a lot of creativity they can make a beautiful form of decoration for their room from a simple leaf.

- **Age:** 3–10 years
- **Number of participants:** at least one
- **Space:** wherever
- **Materials:**
    * dry, nice-sized leaves
    * brush
    * paint
    * colored beads

      * sequins

      * legumes

      * glue

- **Method:** This activity starts on the street. You can take advantage of the walk from school or a stroll through the park so that your child can collect from the ground those nice-sized, dry leaves that they like the most. The older the leaf is, the easier it will be to decorate it.

  Once home, ask him/her to clean the leaf well with a dry cloth. Protect the work zone with old newspapers and put your little artist in a robe that can get dirty. From there, only your imagination is required. He/she can paint the leaf different colors and, once the paint has dried, apply with glue and the help of some eyebrow tweezers the beads or sequins. If you don't have these at home, you can also glue lentils or soybeans. If he/she doesn't like the color of the legume, he/she can paint it different colors and afterward put it on the leaf according to what he/she likes.

Artistic collage

With few materials and a little help, your child can prepare a collage of his/her things that he/she will enjoy using. You can choose a set theme or period of time, like Christmas vacation or summer camp.

- **Age:** 6–12 years
- **Number of participants:** at least one
- **Space:** wherever
- **Materials:**
      * brown paper or cardboard
      * glue
- **Method:** First he/she should decide where the collage will be hung in order to choose the size of the brown paper or cardboard and

the size of the things that he/she is going to glue on it. Once it is cut out, your child can glue the things that he/she likes, like photos or drawings, or make a craft that involves applying a different memento every day for some time. For example, you can choose the theme of vacation and, every day, glue something that you have done: a ticket to the park, train ticket, seashell, photo with friends, etc. The paper can be stuck to one of the walls of the place at which you vacation, and each day add something new. With that, he/she will have a beautiful memory, and if he/she makes it with friends, it will be even more fun.

Face of the plate

When the rain destroys an afternoon at the park, or there is too much time spent being inactive, this simple, fun craft can be a creative, didactic solution. With simple materials, children can create characters that star in puppet shows. The diversion is a certainty and the TV is turned off.

- **Age:** 5–10 years
- **Number of participants:** however many
- **Space:** wherever
- **Materials:**
    * paper or plastic plate
    * remnants of fabric
    * paper
    * yarn
    * a ruler or a stick
    * glue
    * colors or temperas
    * round-pointed scissors

- **Method:** The objective is that the child converts all of those materials into a puppet show. To do so, he/she should draw a face on the plate. He/she can paint the eyes with colors or temperas, or glue on two buttons. He/she can also put on a crumpled paper ball 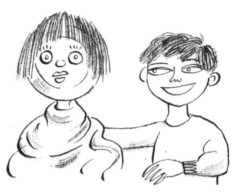 as a nose or a small piece of sponge. Once the face is drawn, he/she can put on hair by gluing threads of yarn or pieces of cotton painted with temperas.

  To create the clothing he/she should cut out a remnant of cloth in the shape of a square or circle and use round-pointed scissors to make a hole in the center.

  Next, he/she has to glue the stick or ruler to the base of the face and pass the clothes via the rod through the hole. Once this operation is done, he/she should glue the clothing to the back of the face. And the puppet is done. He/she can make different ones, such as a princess, a devil, the sun, or a gentleman, and create a witty puppet story with them.

House topography

Your house offers your child many possibilities for discovering new textures and enriching their drawings. Wood, stucco, parquet, tile, rugs . . . they are many and your child probably hasn't paid attention to them until now. And he/she is going to discover them.

- **Age:** 5–10 years
- **Number of participants:** at least one
- **Space:** wherever

- **Materials:**
  - * paper
  - * colored pencils or crayons
- **Method:** The only thing that your child should do is lean the paper on the texture that he/she wants, for example that of the dining room table, and color softly with the colored pencil or the side of a crayon. In this way, he/she will have "drawn" wood, bricks, carpets, floor tiles, or whatever he/she desires.

  It is a good way of providing texture to specific parts of a drawing. If he/she decides to draw a closet, he/she can paint the wooden texture on the doors. The only requirement in order to best appreciate the result is that it is a big drawing.

Sandy landscapes

This craft can be achieved with much or little ability. The most skilled can make a landscape and the smaller ones make a rainbow. The final result is equally pretty and surprising. In addition, it can be converted into a perfect present for a friend or grandmother.

- **Age:** 5–10 years
- **Number of participants:** at least one
- **Space:** wherever
- **Materials:**
  - * sugar or sand
  - * colored chalk
  - * a crystal jar with a lid
  - * cellophane colored paper
  - * elastic band or tie
- **Method:** Kids will enjoy the beauty, reducing the colored chalk to dust, and so it is advisable that you protect them with a robe and the work area with old newspapers. Once the chalk is reduced to

dust, it is mixed with the sugar or fine sand from the beach into mounds separated by color. Afterward, they should pour the colors inside the jar, little by little, forming the art or landscape. In order not to waste so many pieces of chalk, the center of the jar can be filled with sugar without painting, since it will not be seen once it is completed.

When they have finished, they should put a good layer of white glue on top and cover the jar to set the design of colors in the interior. Once the glue has dried, the jar can be manipulated without risking the possibility that the art will be ruined. Now is the time to cut a piece of cellophane paper in a circle bigger than the lid of the jar. They should put it on top and attach it to the "neck" of the jar with the help of an elastic band or a tie. And so, the jar will now be ready.

Gifty postcards

The ideal occasions to give a postcard as a gift are many: birthdays, sacred holidays, wedding anniversaries, and Christmas. Without a doubt, this time not only will he/she write the text, but also he/she will create the postcard itself with it, which that will serve as a personalized gift to delight whoever receives it.

- **Age:** 7–12 years
- **Number of participants:** at least one
- **Space:** wherever
- **Materials:**
    * cardboard
    * pencil
    * colored pencils or markers
    * ruler
    * round-pointed scissors

- **Method:** On a piece of cardboard, draw, in pencil, a rectangle about 12 inches (30 cm) by 8 inches (20 cm). Trace a line 6 inches (15 cm) high to separate the postcard into two halves. Next, cut out the whole rectangle, which will be the base where your child will draw the motif that he/she desires and will write the text.

    Once cut out, the postcard is folded via the line that was previously traced. The outside part is where your child should draw what he/she likes the most on this occasion, like a birthday cake, a present, or a Christmas tree, for example. And the internal part is where he/she can write the text for the recipient of the postcard.

    The possibilities are many because he/she can vary the color of the cardboard or the materials used to draw, so that he/she can create many distinct postcards.

Juggling balls

How many times have we been awestruck watching a performance by a street juggler? Although it can seem to be the contrary, it is easier to make the juggling balls, and then afterward, what requires the most patience is to actually juggle them. With very simple materials and very little help, your kids can make different colored balls and spend the passing hours practicing. It will end up being the newest diversion in your house.

- **Age:** 5–13 years
- **Number of participants:** at least one
- **Space:** wherever
- **Materials:**
    * colored balloons that are not too big
    * little plastic bags or plastic wrap
    * round-pointed scissors
    * rice

- **Method:** The child should cut the "neck" of the balloon in a way so that only the round part is left. Next, he/she should put half a cup of rice in a plastic bag and attach it or wrap it in plastic wrap so it looks like a small ball. Once this is done, the ball is placed inside the balloon, which will stay perfectly tightened. Afterward, another balloon is introduced from the other side and the juggling ball is made.

  To decorate it, he/she can make a third balloon that, previously, will have been pierced with a needle to make a colorful polka-dotted ball.

  He/she can start making two to practice different games and, to the extent that he/she improves, he/she can add new balls to the collection.

Draw with the foot

Kids always like to draw, most typically with their hands. If you propose to your child to draw with his/her foot, you are going to surprise him/her and, in addition, he/she is going to have a lot of fun. All that is needed is his/her foot, a pencil, and paper, so that you can put your feet to work!

- **Age:** 6–10 years
- **Number of participants:** at least one
- **Space:** wherever
- **Materials:**
  * paper
  * pencil
- **Method:** Put a piece of paper on the ground and close to a chair of a height from which your child

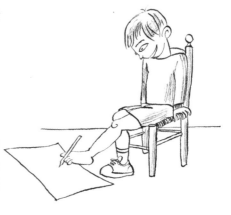

can easily have his/her feet reach the ground. Ask him/her to take off his/her shoes and that he/she holds a pencil between the thumb and index toes. With the pencil, he/she should draw what he/she wants (or can) on the paper. It is a very fun project with surprising results.

Also, he/she can draw the silhouette of his/her other foot or try to write his/her name. If he/she is older he/she can play a guessing game about what he/she has tried to draw, or make an artistic foot-painting competition.

Precious rocks

This is a very appropriate activity for the long summer afternoons, when our kids are on vacation and they don't know what to do with so much free time. Go to the beach or on the mountain, and nature itself will give us the necessary resources to help our kids spend a good time and stimulate their creativity.

- **Age:** 3–10 years
- **Number of participants:** at least one
- **Space:** the park, beach, forest, or your house
- **Materials:**
    * rocks, shells, tree bark . . .
    * a shoe box, or something similar
    * tempera paintings
    * newspaper or old poster
    * brushes
    * remnants of fabric
    * yarn
    * items to decorate, like vegetables, seeds, buttons . . . (optional)
    * glue (optional)

- **Method:** Encourage your child to get a box or a bag and go to the beach or to the forest for a stroll while collecting pretty rocks, pebbles, or shells. Once he/she has them, he/she should wash them well with the help of water, soap, and a scrubber. With that, the rest of the dirt, dust, and sand will be removed in order to be able to stick to the painting and the glue that afterward will be applied on top.

  After covering the work surface and your child, then it is time to paint the materials the color he/she prefers. One can imitate a ladybug using a pebble or paint some shells to make a necklace, imitate a crab, or emulate a fish. To get more realistic effects, use other materials, like yarn to make the crab legs, watermelon seeds to make the small black spots of the ladybug, or a little bit of glitter on top of the paint to create the shine of the jewels. The limit, as always, is your imagination. Remember that before applying the materials he/she should let the paint dry very well, and leave the rocks or shells on top of some old newspapers for a reasonable amount of time.

Decorate your plant pots

When spring is approaching, many windows are full of pretty potted flowers. It is a good moment for your child to put his/her personal touch on your pots and remain entertained for some time while making the drawings that will be printed on them. Thus, your plant pots will look good and your windows will be full of color.

- **Age:** 6–12 years
- **Number of participants:** at least one
- **Space:** wherever
- **Materials:**
    * a clay pot

* potatoes
* brush
* paint
* cookie molds
* knife
* varnish

- **Method:** The first step to decorate a plant pot is to clean it well of dust or dirt with a cloth. Afterward tell your child that he/she will be using the potatoes and the cookie molds to paint the pot. The potatoes should be of a size just bigger than the molds. They should be cut through the middle and stuck on one side of the molds. With a lot of caution, or with your help, your child should eliminate the potato that projects from the mold with the help of a knife, so that the surface of half of the potato has taken the exact shape of the cookie mold.

  Next, cover the work zone with newspapers and protect your child with a robe or an old shirt. Tell him/her to wet the brush with the paint and paint the potato. While they are moist, he/she should apply them on top of the pot so that the chosen image stays well printed.

  Once the paint is dry, he/she can apply a coat of varnish to obtain a prettier final result.

Magazine messages

This project consists of leaving secret messages for friends, siblings, or additional family members in an envelope. Without a doubt, they are very personal messages in the sense that your child should look for the letters in different magazine and old newspaper headlines. The search is very entertaining and the preparation is also, so that the child has already been assured of a good time.

- **Age:** 8–12 years

- **Number of participants:** at least one
- **Space:** wherever
- **Materials:**
  - * magazines and old newspapers
  - * round-pointed scissors
  - * glue
  - * paper
  - * envelope
- **Method:** The child should first write the message on a separate piece of paper and make a list of the letters that he/she needs to find in the titles of magazines and old newspapers. For example, four "e's," three "j's," five "r's," two "a's," etc.

  Next, he/she should go looking for those letters in distinct headlines with different styles and letter sizes. Once he/she has them all, he/she should stick them on the paper to write the secret message. He/she can also put the recipient's name on the envelope.

Variable: This is a very original form of sending letters to friends, or making a postcard to celebrate a birthday, so there are many possibilities.

Easy mobile

The simple and creative activities are ideal for entertaining our children and giving us parents a breather. Certainly, in the house you have some wired hangers, such as one from the dry cleaner, so your little artist can make good use of the hanger and convert it into a work of art—and with the help of only his/her imagination and his/her own hands.

- **Age:** 4–10 years
- **Number of participants:** at least one

- **Space:** wherever
- **Materials:**
    - * a closet hanger
    - * colored paper or clothing pieces
    - * magazine photos of objects or people
    - * glue
    - * drill
    - * round-pointed scissors
    - * thread or string
- **Method:** The child should completely recoat the hanger with the colored paper or the clothing pieces. Afterward, he/she should select from the magazines the images that he/she wants to hang from his/her mobile, like animals, stars, characters, etc. Once chosen, he/she cuts them out and, with the help of the drill, makes a hole very close to the border of the upper part of the figure. Once the hole has been made, he/she should pass the thread or the string through and make a knot. It is advisable to have a different thread or string length for each object so that each will hang at different levels. When all the figures have their strings, he/she can attach them to the base of the hanger.

    Since this mobile is so simple to make, the child can change the objects that hang from it according to his/her interests or tastes, and can even make some to give to a friend as a gift.

Ex libris

Many bookstores, stationery stores, and toy stores sell stamps with initials or simple illustrations to personalize the books. It is enough to choose what the child likes the most, to soak it in ink, and to place it with a light pressure above one of the first sheets of his/her books so the whole world knows who the owner is.

But if you want your child to make his/her own ex libris, he/she needs to design his/her own drawing.

- **Age:** 8–11 years
- **Number of participants:** at least one
- **Space:** wherever
- **Materials:**
  - * small potato
  - * colored temperas
  - * knife
  - * paper napkin
  - * newspapers or plastic
- **Method:** To start, protect the work surface with newspaper or plastic. Tell your children to think about a simple shape, like a star, a heart, a fish, or his/her initial.

  Afterward, he/she should split the potato down the middle and make the image with the point of the knife. With your help, your child can cut the outline of the drawing. This one should be like relief art.

  Next, he/she should place a paper napkin above the image so that it absorbs some of the moisture from the potato. Soak the potato in paint to apply it on the surface of the book page. It is recommended to let it dry to avoid smearing the previous page upon closing the book.

Variable: Instead of a potato he/she can use a cork cap, or a thick laminated sheet that, once cut out, can be glued with superglue on a wooden or plastic base that can handle it.

Animated book

With this craft your child can create his/her own animated drawings. It is not necessary to draw very well or to spend hours tracing the vignettes. All that is needed is to choose a simple motif and to make it move across the pages of a notebook. It seems magical and here we explain to you how to achieve it.

- **Age:** 10–12 years
- **Number of participants:** at least one
- **Space:** wherever
- **Materials:**
  - * plain-covered notebook
  - * marker
- **Method:** The first step is to choose the motif that your child is going to draw. It should be simple, because it will have to be repeated a lot and if it is very involved it will not be fun. For example, it can be a stick figure or a circular face with eyes and a mouth.

  The drawing should be made on a corner of the sheets; it can be whichever one, but the top right makes it easier to show the final product to friends and family afterward. Once the drawing and its position has been chosen, your child should decide what movement he/she wants to create: a doll that dances, a face that smiles and then becomes serious, marbles that fly in the air.

  Next, the method is very simple. He/she should make a drawing on each page, but vary the movement a bit. In other words, if the doll walks, on each page she should advance her leg a bit more. When the whole sequence has been drawn, he/she will have obtained the result of an animated drawing when leafing through the pages very quickly between the thumb and index fingers. He/she can do it in the order in which he/she has drawn it, or in reverse, from back to front. In both cases, it is very fun and seems magical.

Small puzzle

One of the games that entertains the kids the most is solving puzzles. Here we propose that, in addition, you create the puzzle, so the game becomes a project as well. In addition to their observation skills, it also increases their creativity and technical skill.

- **Age:** 8–12 years
- **Number of participants:** at least one
- **Space:** wherever
- **Materials:**
  - * white poster board
  - * pencil
  - * round-pointed scissors
  - * brush
  - * paint
  - * adhesive plastic
- **Method:** To start to make the puzzle, your child should make a big enough drawing on the poster board, like a mushroom or a landscape. Afterward, he/she paints it and, with your help, he/she laminates it with adhesive plastic.

  Afterward, he/she should turn it over to the blank poster board and trace the pieces of the puzzle with a pencil. Next, cut out the pieces, cautiously, and voilà—he/she has finished making the puzzle. Now he/she just has to do it.

Variable: He/she can also create puzzles of color photocopies of some photo that he/she likes, such as a photo with one of his/her classmates, for example. You should ask only for a place that makes you a photocopy (folio size) in color of the photo that the child wants, or print it on your printer if you have it digitized on your computer. The system is very similar, but instead of drawing the motif of the puzzle, he/she only needs to glue the photo on the poster. The rest of the process is identical to that which we explained to you above.

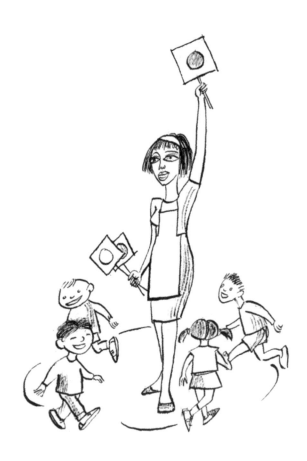

Games to practice inside the house

Traffic light

Road safety is fundamental in the education of our children, and since they were small we taught them to respect the signals and the traffic lights. This game is a good way of practicing these instructions until they become automatic.

- **Age:** 3–10 years
- **Number of participants:** at least four
- **Space:** wherever
- **Materials:**
  - * red and green cardboard
  - * round-pointed scissors
  - * glue or adhesive tape
  - * popsicle sticks, plastic sticks, or pencils
- **Method:** You should ask the children to get in a circle with a separation of 3 ½ feet (1 m) between them at a minimum to avoid having them crash into each other. Next, put yourself, or one of the children, in the center of the circle with cardboard squares of yellow, red, and green. You can glue a stick to each one to convert them to small signs that help drivers.

The children should walk around the circle while you hold up the green sign and repeat, "The traffic light is on green." Without prior warning raise the red sign and indicate, "The light is red." To this order they should all stop short and wait for you to raise the green sign. The children can take turns making the traffic light and you can even include another sign, such as the one-way or dangerous-curves sign.

Three-legged race

This is a traditional game that can be found at many high school parties or summer camp competitions. You can also play this game at home if you have a long hallway in your house or if you can go down to a park.

- **Age:** 8–11 years
- **Number of participants:** at least four
- **Space:** wherever, but a cleared area
- **Materials:**
    * 2 handkerchiefs or cords to attach the legs
- **Method:** It is a very simple game to play. The participants are paired up and the pairs then run as one. This is done by attaching a handkerchief to the left leg of one partner and the right of the other, at the height of the ankle and the knee. This game demands a lot of coordination, since they need to run in a way so that the attached legs act as one. You can make races between various pairs, or time one person if there is not much space. He/she who runs fastest wins. The pair that wins can get a simple prize, like telling a joke; he/she who loses will have to do something tedious, like setting or clearing the table.

Searching for treasure

At times it can seem oppressing to stay in the house on a cold winter afternoon. Without a doubt, all of that changes if you convert the house to a treasure island. With a little imagination, you can get your kids to see their room as part of a treasure map that contains hidden surprises to discover.

- **Age:** 7–12 years
- **Number of participants:** at least one
- **Space:** wherever, even your house
- **Materials:**
    * paper
    * pen
    * a treasure: candy, an allowance, a gift . . .
- **Method:** The first thing to create is the treasure. It doesn't have to be anything spectacular, though, as the important part of this game is the search. Next, you should write some small notes which, through riddles or word games, guide your child toward the treasure. The clues shouldn't be very complicated. It is sufficient to put one in the middle of the dining table, for example, that says something like this: "If you search well in the kitchen, you will be closer to the treasure, pirate!" You need to hide the notes a little only in the rooms that you decide, and you can even include a map with which the child should take steps to find them in one direction or another.

    This game is very entertaining and motivates kids a lot, because it is different from many others. Try it and you will see how your little one asks for it time and again.

Variable: You can create the route with your child, and that can become one of the activities of a birthday party or a reunion with friends. He/she will help you to prepare the marks, to conceive the route, or even to decide on the treasure. It will all be a team effort to pleasantly surprise your child's friends.

Rolling logs

In this game, it is not necessary to have ability or to be fast, or to know how to coordinate your movements too much. You only have to roll and roll . . . It can be a great idea for those difficult afternoons when the kids are fighting, because it will allow them to forget their quarrels and laugh together instead.

- **Age:** 7–12 years
- **Number of participants:** at least three
- **Space:** wherever, but a cleared area
- **Materials:** none
- **Method:** In this game, the logs are their own participants. The kids, and you yourself, if you feel like it, lie facedown on the floor, or on a rug to imitate the logs. One of the participants should serve as a "jockey," but the posture isn't seated, but rather also lying down facedown, perpendicular above the logs, at the height of the backs of their companions. Next, all of the logs start to roll in the same direction. The object is to lead the "jockey" to your liking, at times very quickly, and at others softly. When the horseman has passed the last log, he/she reaches the point where he/she serves as a "rolling" participant and the first in line becomes the new horseman. The game can continue until it arrives at the end of the hall, or the patio—or if it is summer, until you run out of space.

Contortionists

Human contact is always comforting and, in this case, it can also produce a lot of laughter. Intending to maintain original postures with the only parts in contact being your knees, shoulders, and hands is a simple game and also complicated at the same time. It is a fun idea that will promote contact between you and your kids and between your child and his/her friends.

- **Age:** 4–8 years
- **Number of participants:** at least two, in pairs
- **Space:** wherever
- **Materials:** none
- **Method:** Pair up with your child and try to connect the parts of your body with his/hers: your elbows with his/her elbows, your knees with his/hers, the ears, the navels . . . Normally, small kids achieve each contact separately, but to the extent that they grow, they are capable of maintaining two or three contacts at a time, like the shoulders, feet, and hands, for example. With that, and with the height difference between you and your child, you can get very interesting positions and, in doing so, very fun positions.

Uprooting onions

It is a classic game for life that always helps to pass the time when you're waiting or on rainy afternoons. In addition, it teaches the kids to combine forces and play as a collective team and does not encourage competitiveness because no one wins in this game. Although it can seem like a game that's suitable for only wide-open spaces, it can be played without problems in the hall.

- **Age:** 4–12 years
- **Number of participants:** at least four
- **Space:** wherever, but a cleared area
- **Materials:** none
- **Method:** One of the participants is seated supported by a wall, with legs separated and pulled up, and in front of him/her and seated, in an identical position, are the rest of the kids who are participating in the game. They have to squeeze between them all that they can and hug themselves strongly around the waist, in a way that each one

maintains a strong grip around the person in front to form a line of squeezed bodies. They should all sit, except one. The person who stays standing should seize the first in line and intend to pull him/her out of the arms of his/her companion with all his/her strength. When he/she has done so, the person who did the uprooting hugs from behind he/she who has just been taken out of line and the two join forces to uproot the next player in the line of "onions" that are waiting to be seized from the floor.

Card castles

Ability and patience are the keys of this simple game that requires only a plain surface, a deck of cards, and a steady hand. Your child will feel older if you let him/her play a game of adult cards, but he/she can also make castles with whatever childhood deck he/she has amongst his/her toys.

- **Age:** 6–12 years
- **Number of participants:** at least one
- **Space:** a plain surface in a place that is not windy.
- **Materials:**
    * a deck of cards
- **Method:** The best manner of constructing card castles is by joining the top sides of the cards and separating the bottom edges, as if you were making a camping tent. Next you make another at the first one's side, and another, and another. Afterward, horizontal cards are placed over the line that was previously constructed and, next, you return to do the same operation that you did at the beginning. The balance between the cards is the only limit of this game, and your child can create new ways of placing the cards so that he/she keeps increasing his/her ability.

    The castles can have whatever structure the child desires. They can evoke a pyramid or have spaces between the cards simulating windows, or can be a rectangular construction with small "battlements" separated on the last floor, as if it were a medieval wall.

When the castle has been constructed he/she can knock it over with marbles, or intend to have a castle competition with his/her brother or sister, or with a friend.

Cooperative "kidnapping"

Here no one wins and everyone gets to know each other better. It is an ideal strategy for those birthday parties where you have a large mix of school friends, cousins, or siblings, as it is a game that helps everyone get to know each other better and break the ice.

- **Age:** at least six years old
- **Number of participants:** at least six, in pairs
- **Space:** wherever
- **Materials:**
    * pairs of colored handkerchiefs
- **Method:** Ask the kids to cover their eyes with the handkerchiefs. The color that they choose is not important, but you should assure yourself that they don't see anything and that they don't know what colors their companions have chosen. What they know is the color that they themselves have and that another of their friends has the same color.

    Next they should try to test their fellow participants and ask them separately for their tastes and interests. If the interests coincide, then they should ask for the color of the handkerchief and, if it is the same, they can accomplish the "kidnapping." If they don't have the same color handkerchief, the two will be able to continue looking for another participant in the game who shares interests and their same color handkerchief.

Fear of the hat

Kids enjoy having conversations in which they imitate adults. With this game, they will be able to speak of topics that they don't normally address and will help us get to know them better. It is a calm game but a very interesting one and it will help you communicate with your child in a relaxed, fun environment.

- **Age:** at least eight years old
- **Number of participants:** at least two
- **Space:** wherever
- **Materials:**
    * pencils
    * paper
    * a big, opaque container, like a hat or shoe box
- **Method:** Ask all those who participate in the game to sit on the floor in a circle. Next, give each one a small piece of paper and a pencil. On the paper they should write, in an anonymous form, the phrase "I'm afraid of . . ." and whatever they fear. Afterward, they fold the paper well and put it in the hat.

    When all have put their paper inside, shake the hat well and pick one. Read its contents aloud and discuss it amongst everyone. If you prefer, all of them can be read first and then comments can follow at the same time.

Variable: It doesn't necessarily have to be a negative phrase. You can also play by asking about happy things, projects, or interests. You can also put the five things that each one would take from Earth to an imaginary planet's congress or a deserted island. Your tastes and your imagination build the boundary.

The imaginary ball

If your child has ever dreamed of being a juggler, this is a good way to achieve it without risking that the ball falls to the ground. As it is imaginary, the ball will be able to do whatever you please before being thrown to you or one of your friends. It is all a means of entertainment and does not require anything to win the game.

- **Age:** 3–10 years
- **Number of participants:** at least five
- **Space:** wherever
- **Materials:** none
- **Method:** Tell the kids to hold hands and form a circle. Afterward, ask them to drop their hands and, in the same position that they are in, throw, from one person to another, an imaginary ball. The kids can bounce it before tossing it, passing it with their hand, foot, head, or back . . . and receiving it in the same way that it was thrown or whatever way they prefer. The rule is that it can't be thrown two consecutive times in the same way.

> **Variable:** You can also do this game using a balloon instead of a ball, with which the emotion will be heightened, since whoever pops the balloon loses.

A bestial story

Kids love to pretend to be animals and, above all, to imitate them. With this game of imagination, you give them the possibility of creating their own imitations or dying of laughter while you yourself imitate them. Thus they will strengthen their ability to integrate in the group, their ability as mimes, and their imagination. Be careful, it can hook them.

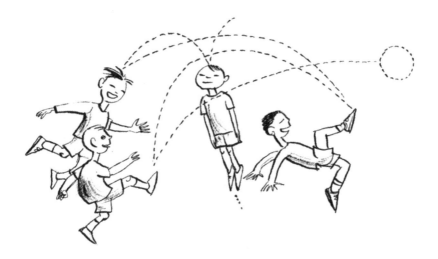

- **Age:** 4–7 years
- **Number of participants:** at least two
- **Space:** wherever
- **Materials:** none
- **Method:** The only thing that should be done in this game is to look for a story or fable in which animals appear. If you don't have anything in the house, don't worry, you can invent your own story, which will increase the excitement. Your child, or a friend, or both, should imitate the movements and the sound that each of the animals that appear in the story emits. If you prefer, they can invent the fable and you can be the one to imitate the animals. It will surely be a good way to get them to continue laughing like never before and so that they will want to be relieved after.

Pin the tail on the donkey

This game is very simple to achieve and the kids love it. You can do it wherever and with whatever material, with your child or with all their friends. In addition, it doesn't necessarily have to be a donkey—you can change the animals and the objects to hang: a chicken and the crest, an elephant and the tusks, a dinosaur and the tail, etc.

- **Age:** at least six years old
- **Number of participants:** at least four
- **Space:** wherever
- **Materials:**
  - * a chalkboard or big poster board
  - * a rope or something similar
  - * adhesive tape to stick the tail, or a magnet if the chalkboard is magnetic
  - * a handkerchief to cover the eyes
- **Method:** On the chalkboard or poster board you should draw a donkey, but without the tail. The game consists precisely of this: pinning the tail on the donkey. The tail can be made with some long material, like a rope, a handkerchief, or a bunch of pieces of wool with a knot. You should look for something strong enough to hang from the drawing based on the chalkboard or poster board that you have chosen.

  To hang the donkey's tail, choose the lucky participant who will be in the first spot. Once chosen, you should blindfold him/ her with the handkerchief and give him/her some turns so that he/ she is a little disoriented. At that point he/she should be focused on the indications of his/her friends, who should guide him/her to be in front of the chalkboard. Next, with orders like up, down, right, or left, they should indicate to the player where to pin the tail on the donkey to complete the drawing.

Variable: If you are a big group, you can draw many donkeys and form the same number of teams. The kids chosen to put the tail on the donkey of their team will have to pin it at the same time, which will create jubilation for all the groups giving instructions at the same time.

Submarine

We have all seen some movies where a submarine navigates through the depths and, at some moment, emits the signal of a sharp whistle. This game evokes that action in a certain way, but those who whistle are the players in the game, and he/she who "navigates" (the one crawling) is your child.

- **Age:** 6–10 years
- **Number of participants:** at least four
- **Space:** wherever
- **Materials:**
   * handkerchief to cover the eyes
- **Method:** Tell all the participants to be seated on the floor approximately 3 ½ feet (1 m) apart. Choose one of the players to cover his/her eyes and, next, this one should pass like a cat through the rest of the players who are seated. When some of the players see that the submarine, that is, he/she who crawls with covered eyes, is about to bump into them, they should rapidly emit a whistle (piii, piii!) or whatever other signal they have previously established to advise their partner that he/she should switch routes to avoid a crash.

Variable: It is a game that allows many variables, as it can be played with various submarines: add new obstacles like a set signal for each one of them, distribute small prizes throughout the game room, etc.

A lemon and a half

This simple game of attention and reflexes usually provokes with ease the laughter of whoever is participating. Although we propose this phrase, it can be whichever one you can invent; whichever player is called decides.

- **Age:** 8–11 years
- **Number of participants:** at least five
- **Space:** wherever
- **Materials:** none
- **Method:** Seat the kids in a line and assign each one a number. The number one should start saying, as quickly as possible, "A lemon and a half calling to five and a half lemons," for example. Then the person that has number five should do the same, but say, "Five and a half lemons calling three and a half lemons." Each child announced by their number should, on his/her turn, call the other. And it goes on like this successively. As they will repeat it very rapidly and they have to be very attentive, the errors start to appear, and with them the laughter, above all if the parent is the one who makes the mistake.

> **Variable:** In the moment of saying the phrase, the player should put his/her hands on his/her temples and flap them like insect antennae. In addition, he/she who is to the right should put his/her left hand on his/her temple, and he/she who is to the left of the person saying the phrase will be able to put his/her right hand on his/her temple.

Ping-pong cups

With very simple elements, your child and you can create a game in which the kids will believe they are shooting cans with balls as they would at the fair. If you prefer to apply the variable of applying actions instead of points to the cups, the game is converted to a fun succession of somersaults, jokes, or hugs, which limits the competitiveness and adds fun.

- **Age:** 9–11 years
- **Number of participants:** at least four
- **Space:** wherever
- **Materials:**
  - * 20 small plastic cups
  - * 3 ping-pong balls
  - * paper
  - * pencil
- **Method:** Place the plastic cups on the table. Previously you should label some small paper boxes with the numbers one through three. You should place these papers under the cups and each will be the score that each cup will have. If you have permanent markers you can also write the number directly on the cup.

  From a certain distance the participants should throw the three ping-pong balls on each turn and intend to knock down the cups. To avoid having the ball be knocked down by the cups you can establish the rule that it should bounce on the floor before jumping toward the table. Once the three balls are thrown, the total score is noted on a piece of paper.

Variable: This game has a certain competitive air, but you can change the cause of winning to something different, like making the winner tell a joke, or instead of keeping score, writing an action on each small piece of paper, like doing a somersault, winking, or giving a hug.

Spaghetti

The simplest materials often offer us big opportunities to entertain. With this game, your child will develop his/her skill, ability, and, above all, his/her patience to dissolve the knots and tangles that he/she and his/her friends have made. It is a race against the clock so as not to lose an article, and a good excuse to share laughs with friends.

- **Age:** 7–10 years
- **Number of participants:** two to ten
- **Space:** wherever
- **Materials:**
    * a cord of average thickness with about 31 ½ inches (80 cm) in length for each player
    * a stopwatch or clock with a second hand
- **Method:** This game consists of being able to untangle the cord before the rest of the participants. You should have in your hand a stopwatch or a clock with a second hand and a practicing referee. Upon your signal, your little one and his/her friends should focus on tying and messing up the cord the best that they can. After thirty seconds you give a new signal so the first player stops tangling the cord. Next, he/she runs the tangled cord to the friend-opponent to his/her right, who should continue the task of tangling and making knots in the cord that he/she just had passed to him/her. Every fifteen seconds you give a new signal, for as many parts of the game that there are. After you order, "Untangle!" all should hasten the untangling of the cord that they have in their hands at that moment. He/she who first untangles the cord will be the winner. If you want to make the game more interesting, you can ask for a token from the last-place finisher.

The current

In this game various components are needed, but it doesn't require any type of preparation or material. It is easy and very entertaining, so your kids and their friends can have a good time using the help of only their hands and their observation capabilities. If you feel nostalgic of your afternoons as a girl or boy, this is the moment to include yourself in the group and pass the current.

- **Age:** 6–10 years
- **Number of participants:** at least five
- **Space:** wherever
- **Materials:** none
- **Method:** To be able to play, the participants should sit separately forming a circle and taking each other's hands. He/she who stops it should be in the middle. One of the members performs the functions of "central electricity"; that is to say, he/she initiates a "discharge" with a light squeeze of the hands that passes from one to the other. The current can turn or change feeling, in terms of what the player who in the moment is passing it wants. The player who is seated in the center should watch attentively the hands of those who form the circle and intend to guess on which point of the circle the current is located in that moment or, if that is the same, what hand it is that is pressing lightly on that of a friend. If he/she gets it right, the player who passed the current in that moment goes to the center of the circle and he/she who guesses it is incorporated into the circle to pass the current.

The small pig

Performing as the small pig has never been clean or fun. In this simple game, the participants only need to imitate the noise of a pig, and it will leave them laughing. It is very easy and entertaining, and the participants don't like to stop playing.

- **Age:** at least six years old
- **Number of participants:** at least five
- **Space:** wherever
- **Materials:** none
- **Method:** In this game, he/she who seeks should have his/her eyes

well covered. Next, his/her friends are distributed throughout the room silently, and without moving, wait for their friend with the eyes covered to locate them. When he/she who seeks finds one of the participants, he/she should sit cautiously on his/her side, or on his/her knees, and emit the noise of a piglet. The other player should respond in identical form and he/she who seeks should guess by the noise and the sound of the snorting player who he/she is. If he/she gets it right, the person who has been discovered becomes the person with his/her eyes covered, but if the response is incorrect, he/she will be able to look for a new friend and should intend to discover who he/she is. He/she can't touch and the only information that will be provided is the sound.

Musical chairs

It is a classic assembly game that used to entertain courts centuries ago. It does not only entertain kids, but older people participate as well, legend has it. You need only some chairs and a plan to have a good time.

- **Age:** at least four years old
- **Number of participants:** at least five
- **Space:** wherever, but a cleared area
- **Materials:**
  * as many chairs as participants, less one
  * music (radio, CD, an instrument, or, simply, handclaps)
- **Method:** Place in a circle as many chairs as participants, less one, in the center of the space in which you've decided to play. Next, the players are lined up and wait to hear the music, or the sound of the handclaps, to begin to walk or dance around the chairs. When the music stops, everyone should look for a chair in which to sit. The player still standing is eliminated.

Before resuming the music you should take away a chair and continue with the game. And do that successively until there are only one chair and two players left. It will be the final round that will decide who is the winner.

The pickpocketers

With this game we aren't trying to make your child a skillful pickpocketer with dark motives. The only objective is to show that any excuse is good to have a good time. He/she will have never enjoyed the silence so much and you will be relaxed playing.

- **Age:** 7–12 years
- **Number of participants:** at least two
- **Space:** wherever
- **Materials:**
    * a coat
    * a wallet or some keys
    * bells
    * safety pins
- **Method:** With the help of the pins, place various bells on the sleeves, collar, lapels, or tails of a coat that you should hang on a hanger or the back of a chair. Ask the rest of the participants to hide in whichever of the coat pockets the object that you have chosen, or various objects; they can be some keys, a wallet, or even a ping-pong ball.

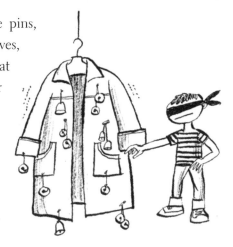

The player who should look for the object indicated by the rest of the participants, and no other, has to find it with his/her eyes covered and without making the bells in the jacket make noise.

If he/she can't achieve it, he/she pays a collateral, although you can also assign a point for each minute that he/she spends and two points for each fault committed upon making the bells make noise. At the end of the game the person with the fewest points or he/she who has conserved the most collateral wins.

The radar

Your grandfather's old alarm clock is a good excuse to test your child's sense of orientation and hearing. With a little imagination and plans to have a good time, you can develop a game of radar.

- **Age:** 6–11 years
- **Number of participants:** at least four
- **Space:** wherever
- **Materials:**
  * handkerchiefs to cover the participants' eyes
  * a bigger handkerchief or scarf
  * an alarm clock that goes "ticktock"
- **Method:** Ask four kids to be placed at the four corners of whichever room, but one that is cleared in the middle. When they are placed, cover all their eyes and put in the middle of the room an alarm clock that goes "ticktock" and, at a little distance from it, a big handkerchief or scarf. Next, the four kids should look for that handkerchief, guiding themselves by the sound of the clock, but without touching it.

Variable: You can make two teams and put two alarm clocks with two handkerchiefs to see who gets away with both handkerchiefs.

Telephone

This game shows kids that whispering transforms information, and how. They will confirm that the same sentence, repeated in a soft voice into the ear, needs only five or six repetitions to transform into a new and crazy sentence. The result is usually hilarious and the dynamic of the game is relaxed and calm, so it's ideal for neutralizing moments of "child chaos."

- **Age:** 8–11 years
- **Number of participants:** at least five
- **Space:** wherever
- **Materials:** none
- **Method:** Place the kids in a circle. One of them should make up a simple sentence, such as, for example, "The other day I went to buy potatoes at the supermarket." Next, he/she should say it into the ear of the person sitting next to him/her and try to prevent the rest of the group from hearing it. This is repeated to the person next to that one, and so on and so forth. When it arrives at the player who initiated the round, this person should say the phrase out loud that he/she has heard and also repeat the sentence that he/she originally made up. The two sentences are usually different and the result is very funny.

The ping-pong ball

This game is very fun because it is easy and thrilling. Without a doubt, it is best for there not to be any really long games so as not to get sick as a consequence of the continuous blasts. The obstacles against those who hit the ball, or for those who have to pass, increase the difficulty and strengthen the ability, speeds, and reflexes of the kids.

- **Age:** at least eight years old
- **Number of participants:** at least two

- **Space:** a table
- **Materials:**
    * a ping-pong ball
    * a table
    * different objects to make obstacles
- **Method:** Each participant is put on opposite sides of the table. The game consists of advancing the ping-pong ball to your opponent's side and getting it to fall to the floor from strong blowing. He/she who defends his/her camp can blow to defend his/her territory. The game becomes more exciting if obstacles are placed to make it difficult to advance the ball, like books or, simply, a glass. They can also create points at which to pass, or create circuits, or even make games of doubles. The referee will keep score to decide who wins the "game."

Mini golf course

Kids love to play mini golf, but it isn't often that you find a course close to home and, also, they are usually tired before finishing the round. This improvised mini golf can give your child the opportunity to have a fun time.

- **Age:** 6–12 years
- **Number of participants:** at least one
- **Space:** a very smooth surface
- **Materials:**
    * coffee cups
    * soup spoon
    * ping-pong balls or wads of aluminum foil
- **Method:** To create the mini golf course, various options exist. You can draw it on a smooth surface, like cardboard or the bottom side of one of those plastic chairs that have roads and blocks drawn on

them. In the latter case it is better to use a permanent marker so it doesn't leave marks on the floor when you turn it over so your child can play with the cars.

If you prefer, mark the course with adhesive tape directly over the floor of his/her room or, simply, don't trace any course. Next, distribute the coffee cups in a horizontal position, like golf holes, at the length of the course.

After deciding which is the exit and which is the goal, your child can start to push the ping-pong ball with the help of the spoon to get it in the "holes." If you don't have ping-pong balls at home, you can improvise a ball with a wad of aluminum foil. It's simple and effective.

Sock dolls

This game is comprised of two phases—one in which the child makes the dolls or characters, and the other in which he/she plays to make stories with them. It is a good way of recycling old or unmatched socks that are always around the house and increasing your child's creativity and imagination.

- **Age:** 8–12 years
- **Number of participants:** at least two
- **Space:** wherever
- **Materials:**
  * old or unmatched socks
  * sewing needle without a point
  * thread
  * colored buttons
  * glue
  * colored yarn
  * markers

- **Method:** This game teaches your child how to turn an old sock into a fun puppet show. He/she can be a princess with long hair or a demon with big fangs, or even the cookie monster. He/she doesn't need a story or script to decide what characters to create, since it is more fun to make the puppet show out of the crazy characters that the hands of your little rascals can create.

  The head of the puppet is the part where the toes go in the sock. On the end he/she can sew or glue colored wool or cotton or whatever material you find around the house. Afterward, on the instep of the sock, draw the face with the markers, or glue buttons as eyes and a cutout piece of cloth as a mouth. If your child likes crafts, he/she can use cardboard covered in aluminum foil to create a king's crown or a magician's hat. As you can see, the possibilities are numerous. When the puppet is finally created, the sock is put on from the hand to the forearm and, with the help of the fingers, the character's movements are simulated. To improvise a small theater, you can cover the table with a blanket and make the characters appear from behind. Thus, he who manipulates them stays hidden and only the movement of the puppets is seen.

> **Variable:** If your child is small, he/she will love that you are speaking through a puppet with these characteristics. You might be really surprised in the case that kids from two to four years old have made the doll that your hand is acting out. Create one and give it a fun name: it will be your best ally for convincing your little one that it is bath time or time to go to sleep.

Find your partner

In this game the kids should write, be fast, and, above all, learn to lose. It is fun and simple to practice, and you hardly need materials. The variables can be many, like joining numbers instead of making pairs or making drawings instead of writing names. Between the preparation and the game, good leisure time will have passed without your even having realized it.

- **Age:** 8–10 years
- **Number of participants:** at least four
- **Space:** wherever, but a cleared area
- **Materials:**
    * a chair for the player
    * paper
    * pencil
    * whistle
- **Method:** The kids should cut out four squares of paper for each player and write on each one half of a pair: for example, Zipi and Zape, dog and cat, police and thief, etc. Next, they should leave in two bowls or whichever other container each one of the parts of the pair that they have created, so that all the pairs of nouns are separated.

    The referee will place throughout the hall, or the place that you have chosen to play in, as many chairs as participants, and he/she will leave on each one of them one of the papers from the bowl that he/she chooses, until having distributed them all.

    The kids will be able to take one of the remaining papers from the bowl. Once the pair that they should look for is known, the referee will whistle to signal the beginning of the game and the kids will go running to look for their pair on each one of the chairs. When they find it, they should conserve the two papers and sit on the seats. The last one to sit loses.

Variable: You can also make the winner be the person who has the least points in various rounds, and in this way you can prolong the game and give each child a chance.

The dancing potato

At times, the imagination is the best weapon to combat the laziness of sitting in front of the TV without any other worry. A simple potato can convert whatever afternoon into an unforgettable time, a product of the laughter that provokes this simple game. All that is needed is coordination and the feeling of rhythm.

- **Age:** 8–10 years
- **Number of participants:** at least four
- **Space:** wherever
- **Materials:**
    * a medium-sized potato
    * music
- **Method:** It is a game that requires coordination and a lot of concentration, but that does not require other material aside from the potato and that is very simple to execute.

    The kids should group together in pairs and, at their turn or all at once, they should place the potato between the cheeks of each one of the constituents of the pair, in a way that it doesn't fall to the floor.

    Next, put on music so that they follow the rhythm, dancing and maintaining at the same time the potato between the cheeks of them and their dance partners. It is evident that he/she who sustains the potato for the longest time wins, although you can also invent categories of prizes, like he/she who dances the best. If a pair dances for such a long time that it does get boring, it could still ultimately make them laugh.

Balloon

Balloons are always present at birthday parties and many of your child's fun times. They can also allow your kids to have a good time and lose their fear of balloons exploding via this improvised game.

- **Age:** 6–11 years
- **Number of participants:** at least five
- **Space:** wherever
- **Materials:**
    * a balloon
    * paper
    * markers
- **Method:** Seat the kids in a circle and let them choose a number between one and five (or more, if there are more participants). To that effect, you can include another game of those we propose to you, like "Rock, paper, or scissors," for example.

    Once each one has been assigned a number, distribute a piece of paper and a marker to each one so that they all write the number, largely. Next, fasten it on the front part of the shirt so that it is clear to all which is his/her number and that of their friends.

    Then, choose at random a number from all those who participate and the child who has that number sits in the center and starts to fill the balloon as much as he/she can with one breath. Once done, choose another number to go to the center, to blow up the balloon once again and to choose a new friend to continue the blowing up of the balloon. You can agree before starting if the person who makes the balloon explode is the one who wins or loses.

Variable: You can also form various teams and have them compete to see whose balloon explodes first. In that case it is not necessary to number the participants; it will work for them to follow the ticking of the clock.

Memory

The game of Memory strengthens the ability of observation, that of retention, and the reflexes of the child. In that which we propose to you, in addition, your child will be able to display his/her artistic qualities and dedicate a good time to "making" his/her own personalized game. To that effect, the time dedicated to entertainment and fun increases and is enriched.

- **Age:** 6–10 years
- **Number of participants:** at least one
- **Space:** wherever
- **Materials:**
  - * poster board
  - * markers
  - * round-pointed scissors
- **Method:** Trace on a poster board a grid with lines separated every 2 inches (5 cm). When you have drawn it, ask your child to cut it out until he/she has obtained squares. Once cut out, he/she should choose a series of drawings that he/she likes, like geometric figures, faces with expressions, numbers, etc., that are easy to make. There should be a total equivalent to half the squares cut, so that he/she can draw a pair of each. With the help of colored markers and a little patience, he/she will be creating a personalized game of Memory.

  Once he/she has drawn the squares, they are mixed facedown and are distributed on a table or simply on top of the rug. Next, he/she should turn them over two by two and intend to find the pairs. He/she can play alone or against another participant. He/she who finds the most pairs when the squares have all been turned over wins.

Change of clothes

Each morning it is a triumph for our kids to get dressed quickly. Without a doubt, this game will produce authentic miracles and kids will undress and dress at lightning speed. The results are usually worthy of a funny photograph for the family album and the kids have a great time.

- **Age:** at least six years old
- **Number of participants:** at least four
- **Space:** wherever
- **Materials:**
  * the clothes that they have put on or costumes
- **Method:** Kids should form two teams with a minimum of two players each to compete in a wardrobe race against the clock. The idea is that they are entertained simply with the clothes they have on. It is evident that if you propose this game to them in the winter they should do it in a heated room. If you take this precaution, it is the ideal time to play the clothes-changing game, since they wear a lot more garments in the winter than in the summer. The game consists of the players from each team undressing completely and then dressing with the garments in reverse in the least amount of time possible. In other words, first the jersey, then the shirt, and lastly the T-shirt, or first the pants and after the underpants. It is a manner of dressing contrary to the usual way and with which truly crazy results are obtained.

Variable: Instead of dressing in the opposite order, they can put on the clothes inside out—in other words, seam out—or interchange clothes with the members of the opposite team. This last variable is very fun, although it is advisable that the participants have a similar physical physique, or else it's not fun.

Small theater

Parents, family, and friends will be a part of the "public" that will see this work of theater, although another fun form of onstage work exists: making use of a video camera fastened to a tripod to tape the performance. Thus the kids themselves will be able to make a movie that will delight all when it is shown on the TV. In this case, the TV will come to be their method of expression rather than a passive game.

- **Age:** 8–11 years
- **Number of participants:** at least two
- **Space:** wherever
- **Materials:**
  - * a pencil
  - * pieces of paper
  - * old clothes, costumes
  - * makeup
- **Method:** The kids should think about a story or problem, some characters, the setting of the work, and the wardrobe that they are going to need. They can first look for the clothes for inspiration and, from then on, create the text. On the paper they shouldn't only write the dialogues, but rather also they should note the gestures and actions that accompany the text.

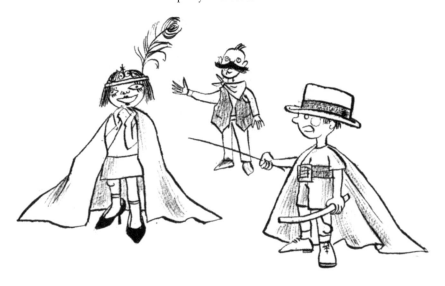

When they have written the "mini-book," the time to get dressed up and put on makeup arrives for the onstage work. They can look around the house for objects with which to create a set to give more veracity to the work. And, after a few rehearsals, they can become authentic actors.

Fishing

This one is a very fun game that requires the participation and creativity of the child, so that, in addition, it is a craft. While he/she prepares it he/she will be well entertained and, once finished, can pass the empty hours fishing for the silver fish that he/she will have created by himself/herself. If it is summer, the game has the fun incentive of refreshing the feet along with the fish inside the bucket, of course, if and when he/she plays on the terrace or the patio.

- **Age:** 5–10 years
- **Number of participants:** at least one
- **Space:** inside the house, on the patio, in the garden
- **Materials:**
    * colored poster board
    * self-adhesive paper
    * clips
    * magnets
    * wooden spoon
    * cord
    * round-pointed scissors
    * a bucket
- **Method:** The first thing that the child should do is make the fish. Depending on the age of the little one, he/she can do it alone, although he/she will need your help if he/she is not very skilled with scissors.

Give him/her poster boards of distinct colors and on which he/she will draw fish, stars, and small sea horses about 4 inches (10 cm) in length. The more colors and shapes, the more exotic the fish will be. Once the fish have been cut out, help him/her to cover them with self-adhesive paper to avoid letting the water dissolve them right away.

Once you have covered everything, put on a clip, which we use to fasten sheets on each one of the fish. It is important that the clips are metallic, because the plastic will not stick to the magnet. So that the water doesn't make the clips break free from the fish, he/she can fasten them well with a little adhesive.

Now that he/she has prepared the fish to pour them into the water, it is time to make the fishing rod. Different methods and materials can be used, although a good idea is to use a wooden spoon, of the kind that has a hole in the handle. Through this hole the cord is passed—you can even use cooking twine—and a strong knot is made. On the other side of the cord, attach a magnet, which will serve as the bait.

Now is the moment of filling a bucket of water, pouring the fish in it, and sitting down to fish. The magnet will be in charge of attracting the metallic clips stuck to the fish and the child will enjoy a fun time fishing.

Variable: If more than one kid participates, a number from one to ten can be noted on the lower part of the fish. When the "fishing" has ended, the score of the capture is noted and the person who has obtained the most points is confirmed.

Secret message

With this game, the child will discover a magic form of sending secret notes with their friends and will leave Grandma open-mouthed. It is a simple chemical experiment, which uses very simple materials, with a surprising result and, in doing so, the child learns about the chemical changes and the oxidation processes of some elements. The child, without help of the adults, will be capable of creating an invisible ink that will be able to reveal itself at will. A little magic will be felt and calligraphy will be practiced without even realizing it.

- **Age:** 5–10 years
- **Number of participants:** however many
- **Space:** wherever
- **Materials:**
    * paper to write on
    * lemon juice or white vinegar
    * a toothpick or a pencil without a point
    * a candle or a lit lightbulb
- **Method:** Put in a glass the white vinegar or juice recently squeezed from a lemon. Afterward, make the child wet the toothpick or the point-less pencil in the liquid and write or draw what he/she wants on the paper. He/she should often wet the point so that the whole sketch is well coated with the juice or vinegar. If he/she wants to improve what he/she is drawing, he/she can place the paper on the crystal of the window to see the wet lines that he/she is making. Once the liquid has dried, what is written disappears and becomes invisible. The process of drying should be natural; if it is helped by a hair dryer or the action of an external source of heat, the second part of this game won't work.

    When the paper is completely dry, help your child get close to a source of heat, which can be a candle, a hot iron, or a lightbulb that has been lit for a few minutes. You should proceed with caution so as not to burn the paper. Once the heat oxidizes the lemon juice or the white vinegar, the drawing that the child has made returns in limited time in a dark tone, a product of the oxidation of the liquid used, and starts to disappear once the heat stops being applied.

Small shop

One of the most entertaining activities for kids is to play store. Hours can be spent selling and buying, as if imitating their elders when they go to the supermarket. Without a doubt, the game can become more attractive, and creative, if they are obliged to create their own store and get articles to sell from all around the house. It is even probable that they will enjoy setting up the store even more than selling or buying.

- **Age:** 4–10 years
- **Number of participants:** at least two
- **Space:** wherever
- **Materials:**
    * a chair or some other surface
    * packages of products and other objects like toys, magazines, or discs
    * marker
    * small sheets to write prices
    * calculator
    * shopkeeper costume (an apron or a painted mustache)
- **Method:** Help your child make a supply of packages and other objects that can serve to play store. Gather them and put them on a table. Help him/her think about the price for each object. The child can write the prices directly on the products or make small signs on sheets. Some can be put on special offer. Once the installation of the store is done, you can play to exchange the shopkeeper and client roles.

  Now you are the client and your child is the cashier. Your child can use the calculator to figure out the checks; he/she will need your help to discover each operation and the corresponding symbols (+, -, ÷, x, y, =), but you can give him/her clues to try to let him/her do it himself/herself.

During the shop game, you can ask questions like, "How much will it cost if I buy three-dozen eggs?" or "How much is a carton of milk worth if the offer is two for $4?" or "How much would the total bill be if I don't buy cereal?" or "How much does my bill increase if I include this magazine?" You can also ask your child to tell you the approximate value of your purchase and afterward confirm it on the calculator.

Marbles

They are the childhood game par excellence and, every now and then, come back in style. Our grandparents played with them, and, surely, our grandchildren will do so, but it is always good to remember when resources are low. Like in some other games, the simplicity is what triumphs.

- **Age:** 6–12 years
- **Number of participants:** at least two
- **Space:** the park or the rug of the dining room (to soften the noise and avoid neighbors complaining)
- **Materials:**
  - * crystal, metal, or whatever other kinds of marbles
- **Method:** Because of the unique characteristics of this game that is well known by all, we will cover only three of the most common variations of the game, as there are so many and it would be too difficult to discuss the many variations that exist.
  - ○ **The bomber:** It is an easy and entertaining variable, great for the smallest ones. A circle of about 12 inches (30 cm) is traced on the floor and each one of the participants places the same number of marbles in the center (two, three, four . . .). Order of turns is determined and the game is begun with the objective to shell the marbles grouped in the circle. The marbles that

leave the circle upon receiving the impact will come to be the property of the player who launched this throw. The game ends when the circle is empty.

○ **The circle:** It is the best known and possibly the oldest of the marble games. Many varieties exist, but the basic method used consists of tracing two circles: one to determine the position of the thrower and the other in which the marbles are found (same amount for each participant). Each player throws a marble with the intention of hitting some of them from the interior of the circle. If he/she gets a marble, it is his/hers. The most experienced players prefer to continue throwing while they hit something on the throw, always with the same marble and from the point at which the marble was after the impact with the other. Another option, fairer for beginners, consists of assigning one throw for each player.

○ **The tunnel:** Consists of introducing the marble from a set distance through a hole or tunnel. As many players as you want can participate. The games can be played in a previously set amount of time or by the number of marbles to throw. Similarly, one or various tunnels of different sizes can be set up and, consequently, differently scored. It all will depend on the wit of the players. A simple shoe box can be cut until four or five holes of distinct sizes are made. That way it is easy.

Add and cross out

This simple game consists of two parts. One is more creative, in which the child is entertained by making six cards that compose it, and another is more educational, in which he/she puts into practice his/her capability of mental calculation. At the end of the game, they will have had a good time and, in the process, will have refreshed their math skills.

- **Age:** 6–10 years
- **Number of participants:** at least two
- **Space:** wherever
- **Materials:**
  - * poster board
  - * square papers
  - * pencil
  - * colored pencils or crayons
- **Method:** The child should make with the poster board some cards with a number on each one from one to six. Once the cards are made, each player should write on a square sheet a series of numbers from one to twelve.

  The cards are shuffled facedown and each player chooses two per turn. Each player should cross out the summations of each of the numbers they draw, in addition to the individual numbers on the cards themselves. If nothing can be crossed out, he/she loses the turn. The player who crosses out all the numbers of their list first is the winner.

> **Variable:** Various rules can be chosen to cross out the numbers from the list. For example, if a five and a six are taken out, the eleven can be crossed out. But also two or three numbers from the list can be crossed out that add to eleven, such as five and six; seven and four; eight and three; nine and two; ten and one; or a combination such as one, two, and eight.

Blind hen

This traditional game is the king of birthdays, but it can also help a child pass a rainy afternoon or play with father and mother. Touch, sound, and orientation are the tools used by the one who is "it," and a costume, wit, and self-control are used by those who are avoiding capture.

- **Age:** 3–10 years
- **Number of participants:** at least three
- **Space:** wherever, but a cleared area
- **Materials:**
  * a handkerchief or something similar to cover the eyes
- **Method:** The more players who participate, the better. The players, holding hands, form a circle. The first seeker is placed in the center of the circle with his/her eyes covered, and has to do all that is possible to trap someone and discover that person's identity.

  The rest of the players go around the circle, bend down, shift, etc. to make the work of the person who seeks difficult in terms of his/her intent to trap them. Given that his/her eyes are closed, he/she who seeks has to find a way to discover the player who has been seized. He/she can use touch, he/she can try to make the player laugh, etc., in order to identify his/her voice, etc.

  On the contrary, when a player is going to be inspected by the person who is "it," he/she can put on a friend's glasses, or a bracelet, etc., to divert them. If he/she who seeks figures out the identity of the player who has been trapped, that person will be the next seeker; if he/she doesn't figure out the identity, that person will have to seek once again.

Rock, paper, or scissors

This simple game has the great advantage of the fact that the "toys" are incorporated into our hands and it serves to have a good time, especially if you're playing to decide who cleans the kitchen or who will go into the bath first. They can also make competitions with the goal of winning more times than the opponent.

- **Age:** at least five years old
- **Number of participants:** two
- **Space:** wherever

- **Materials:** none
- **Method:** The two players are put one in front of the other, and each placing his/her hand behind his/her back, he/she says, "Rock, paper, or scissors." Right at the end of saying the phrase, the two show a hand at the same time and compare the figure or sign that they have chosen.

  They can represent "rock" with the hand closed in the shape of a fist, "paper" if they show the hand flat, and "scissors" if they form the sign of victory with the index and ring fingers.

  The "rock" beats "scissors" because it breaks them, and loses to the "paper" because this can cover it. The "scissors" beat the paper because they can cut it, and they lose to the "rock" because it breaks them. The "paper" beats the rock because it covers it, and it loses to the "scissors" because they cut it.

  If the two players coincide in showing the same figure, the round is annulled, and it doesn't result in points for anyone. A set number of points can be established so that the first person to reach that number wins.

> **Variable:** They can also organize, by the same process explained above, teams that face each other, with a sole participant for each turn. The team that has all its players eliminated first loses.

Bottle caps

Traditionally, it is one of the most popular games. Simply executed and of a peculiar technique, it has brought to life true champions, and its practice allows time to pass at lightning speed. Thus, don't throw away the bottle caps from drinks because they can help bring you more than one afternoon of diversion and laughs.

- **Age:** 5–12 years

- **Number of participants:** at least two
- **Space:** wherever, but a cleared space
- **Materials:**
  * bottle caps
  * Play-Doh
- **Method:** In the first place, it is helpful to fill the caps with Play-Doh so that they weigh a little more and can be managed better.

  It is not advisable for many players to participate, as this contributes to crowding of the bottle caps in the track that is designated. The optimal number of participants is from four to ten.

  On the ground or floor, mark an area, with the help of a stick or chalk, with some stretches of straight lines and curves, of about 10–13 feet (3 or 4 m) long, and about 6 inches (15 cm) wide. Mark an exit line and an entrance line. After figuring out the order of exit, the players, one by one, should propel their bottle caps, helping themselves with the thumb and index finger, so that they are able to send the bottle cap as far as possible, but without leaving the marked area, since this means having to go back to the exit line.

  It is important to procure the ability to not touch the bottle cap of another player, since that advances your rival's cap, and impedes the progress of your own.

Costumes

There is no diversion that equals that of dressing up in costume. It is a creative, fun, and, above all, entertaining activity. Money isn't wasted on buying costumes, as your child would surely like to dress up in his/her father's clothes or with whatever old articles are lying around the house. If you dress up with him/her, the fun will be doubled.

- **Age:** 2–10 years

- **Number of participants:** however many
- **Space:** wherever
- **Materials:**
  - * old clothes
  - * garbage bags
  - * aluminum foil
  - * poster board
  - * tape
  - * round-pointed scissors
  - * wigs
  - * wool, etc.
- **Method:** Although it's not treated as a game, the truth is that it is an activity that entertains and awakens kids' imaginations. You don't have to buy anything, or sew, or be a great designer. On occasion, it will be the child himself/herself who takes the initiative and will surprise you with original ideas. If you both dress up it will be even more fun.

  Here are some ideas to maximize the possibilities of dressing up in the house.

  - ○ **Garbage bags:** They can help your child have a lot of fun. They cover the child's body almost completely and come in different colors. Make holes for the head and arms and, with plastic or paper of other colors, and a little glue, add the details that characterize the costume. These resources make it very easy to make animal costumes. With cardboard, they can make butterfly wings and antennae; or a black cone, which together with a broomstick, will make a small witch costume. If the bag is cut at the height of the knees, with black pants, it will be sufficient to paint a mustache, buy a plastic sword, put a hanky on his/her head, and stick the letter Z on his/her chest to have a Zorro as elegant as Antonio Banderas himself.
  - ○ **Aluminum foil:** This can be used to make bracelets or elements

that simulate metal. If they wrap two boxes, one for the head and another for the trunk, a robot can be made. For the biggest box, add to it futuristic elements, like different color paper buttons. For the arms and legs, cylinders of covered cardboard can be made with the same material.

° **Old clothes:** Much of it that is kept in the bottom of the closet is a great costume. Old clothing or rarely worn clothes can be used to make yourself a superhero, elder, clown, hippie, or pirate. Something as simple as a white shirt can be converted into a medical gown or barber gown for a child.

Handkerchief

Summer camps can include this game amongst the leisurely activities. It does not require anything other than participants and a handkerchief, and interest in having a good time.

- **Age:** 6–10 years
- **Number of participants:** five
- **Space:** best in fresh air, although the dining room can also serve if the center is cleared
- **Materials:**
    * a handkerchief
- **Method:** The minimum number needed to be able to play is two players for each one of the two teams and a person who holds the handkerchief; but the more players who participate, the better.

    Two teams are formed with the same number of players on each. In secret, each team assigns a number to each player. If there are ten players on each side, each one will have a number from one to ten.

    Two lines are formed, and between them is placed the player holding the handkerchief and who will be calling out the numbers.

When, for example, he/she calls out three, the two players, one from each line, who have been assigned this number, will leave their lines. Then each will try to quickly catch the handkerchief and try to bring it to his/her side without being caught by his/her opponent. The player who has the handkerchief is kept on a line that divides the game in two camps. It is very frequent that the pair of players arrives at the hanky at the same time. Then, feints of catching it take place, in a way in which if a player pretends to go for it and the other starts to pursue him/her crossing the line, that player who is doing the pursuing will be eliminated.

When a player is eliminated, the number that he/she had been assigned is given to someone else on his/her team, who, naturally, will have to share two numbers. The team that eliminates all of the opposition's team members wins.

Pica-wall

With this traditional game your child will have a good time and also be able to exercise his/her reflexes. He/she can play it whenever, and it doesn't require any preparation or material, which is invaluable in desperate situations, like rainy afternoons when you can't go to the park.

- **Age:** at least five years old
- **Number of participants:** three to ten
- **Space:** a cleared space with a wall
- **Materials:** not needed
- **Method:** Choose a wall and from this, mark a distance of 23–33 feet (7–10 m).

  The player standing is situated facing the wall. The rest are placed forming a line parallel to the wall at the start of the marked zone.

  The game starts and the player who is "it" has the palms of

his/her hands on the wall, at the time that he/she says, "One, two, three, pica-wall!" While he/she does this, the rest of the players approach him/her rapidly, but with precaution so that he/she doesn't see them so, at the end of the sentence, he/she who is "it" spins quickly and if he/she catches someone moving, he/she will make him/her back off to the point of departure.

The game continues in the same way until one of the players has come close enough to the wall to touch the person who is "it," obliging him/her to be "it" again. But if the person who is "it" traps a player before he/she returns to the line of departure, he/she will be the person who is "it" in the next game.

Remote-controlled car

Although the stores are full of sophisticated toys in stacks, he/she can be much more excited by making his/her own remote-controlled car. While he/she creates, he/she is entertained, and the magic of transporting it by his/her own will can give him/her another good time. The materials are, as always, very basic, and the process of creating it, very simple.

- **Age:** 5–10 years
- **Number of participants:** at least one
- **Space:** wherever
- **Materials:**
    * poster board
    * round-pointed scissors
    * magnets
    * colored pencils, crayons, or markers
    * tape
- **Method:** Ask your child to draw a car, or whatever other vehicle he/she desires, on the poster board. Once drawn, he/she should stick, with adhesive or with the help of a piece of tape, one of the magnets

on the bottom part of the car that he/she has created.

Tell him/her to draw a remote on another piece of poster board and to stick the other magnet on the bottom part.

With the remaining poster board, he/she can construct ramps between furniture or a circuit full of curves. Once done, he/she should put the car in the top part of the circuit and the remote at a distance, just underneath. When the remote is placed at a distance, the attraction of both magnets will move the car by the child's will, like magic.

Also he/she can use other surfaces, as long as they are thin, like the crystal of a window or a layer of wood, to favor the effect of the magnets.

Simple kitchen recipes

Napolitana salad

All of us parents wish that our children have a healthy and balanced diet, and this simple recipe is a good example of that. Tomato with cheese is usually a tasty dish for the young and old alike, so your child will enjoy this salad not only while he/she prepares it, but also when he/she has it on his/her plate.

- **Age:** 8–12 years
- **Number of participants:** at least one
- **Space:** kitchen
- **Materials:**
    * 2 big tomatoes for the salad
    * 3 ½ ounces (100 g) of mozzarella cheese
    * black olives
    * olive oil
    * salt
    * oregano
    * cutting board
    * knife
    * dish
- **Method:** Ask your child to wash the tomatoes well. With the help of a board and a knife he/she should cut the tomato into pieces and

put it in the center of the dish. Next he/she can also cut the mozza-rella cheese into pieces and distribute it around the tomato. If your child has a steady hand, he/she can cut the two ingredients in slices and alternate them in concentric circles around the dish.

Once the ingredients have been arranged he/she has to spread around the black olives on top and sprinkle the salad with oregano. If you prefer, you can substitute the oregano with basil or finely chopped mint. Afterward, all that remains is for you to help season it with salt and olive oil.

Fun pizzas

Pizza is one of the dishes that are most pleasing to kids and there are few who will resist pizzas. And they are a good excuse to introduce such ingredients as tofu, which has a bland flavor and is adapted to perfection on whichever dish. It is certain that your child will create the most fun, nutritious pizza that you can imagine.

- **Age:** 6–12 years
- **Number of participants:** at least one
- **Space:** kitchen
- **Materials:**
    * 1 base for pizza
    * ground tomato
    * olive oil
    * grated cheese (best is mozzarella)
    * salt and pepper
    * tofu
    * carrots
    * champignon mushrooms
    * black olives

* oregano
* board on which to cut veggies

- **Method:** Buy some bases for pizza, great fresh or frozen, at your regular establishment. Ask your child to put on an apron, and wash your hands before starting.

 Turn on the oven to 392°F (200°C) while you prepare the pizza. The first thing is to distribute the ground tomato on the whole surface of the base with the help of a spoon. Next, sprinkle the grated cheese and pieces of tofu. And the adventure starts. Ask your child to create a face with the different cut vegetables on the base of the pizza. He/she can use black olives as eyes, a long piece of carrot for the mouth, pieces of tofu for the nose, and two half-slices of zucchini as ears. But this is only an idea, as he/she can create different faces with the ingredients that he/she most enjoys.

 Once all of the ingredients are distributed, he/she should sprinkle the pizza with a little oregano and it is ready for you to put it in the oven for about fifteen minutes. And thus he/she will have prepared his/her preferred dinner with a fun touch.

Traditional tortillas

Tortillas are tasty to many kids and this recipe is a good way of introducing vegetables into their habitual menu. With a little help from you, they will make a tortilla that makes them lick their fingers.

- **Age:** 8–12 years
- **Number of participants:** at least one
- **Space:** kitchen
- **Materials:**
    * 3 eggs
    * sliced potatoes

* pieces of soft green beans
* 1 mature tomato, in pieces
* ⅔ cup (100 g) of peas
* lettuce
* cherry tomatoes
* knife
* pot
* water
* olive oil
* frying pan

• **Method:** Ask your child to wash, peel, and cut the vegetables while you boil water in a pot. Boil in that water the green beans, carrots, and peas for ten minutes.

Next, heat the olive oil in a frying pan and add the sliced potatoes. Let them cook for five minutes, and, next, add the rest of the vegetables and keep a slow fire going until the potato is cooked.

Tell your child to beat the eggs in a bowl. Add a pinch of salt and let him/her pour all the vegetables into the bowl and mix them with the beaten eggs.

Afterward, make the tortilla in a frying pan and ask him/her to adorn it with a little finely chopped lettuce and cherry tomatoes cut through the middle.

Spaghetti with tomato sauce

The king of all preferred food of your child, it is not too tricky for us. If, in addition, he/she cooks it with your help, it will seem like a delicacy to him/her. You can opt for whole-wheat spaghetti and start to introduce this kind of healthy, nutritious pasta into your diet.

• **Age:** 8–12 years

- **Number of participants:** at least one
- **Space:** kitchen
- **Materials:**
    * 8 ½ cups (2 l) of water
    * 8 ½ ounces (250 g) of spaghetti
    * 1 tablespoon of salt
    * 1 onion
    * 3 tablespoons of olive oil
    * ⅖ cup (100 g) of tuna
    * 6 peeled tomatoes
    * 1 teaspoon of oregano
- **Method:** Put the water with the salt to boil in a pot, and tell your child to peel the tomatoes and to dice them into small pieces. Afterward, he/she has to peel an onion and mince it finely in a mincer.

    Pour a little olive oil in a frying pan and ask that he/she pour in the tuna and onion, but when the olive oil is still cold, in order to avoid it splashing. Allow your child to stir the mixture from time to time while it fries on a slow flame. When it is done, he/she should add the diced tomato. Put in the salt and a small amount of sugar to neutralize the acidic flavor of the tomato. Cover the frying pan and let it boil on a slow flame until the sauce is just right.

    Meanwhile, pour the spaghetti into the boiling water and let it cook for about twenty minutes. Drain the noodles well with a little cold water so that they stay loose and tell your child to separate them onto plates. Afterward, he/she should sprinkle, with your supervision, a little oregano and add some spoonfuls of the sauce on top.

Stuffed tomatoes

This dish, fun and simple to make, introduces the cooking world to your little ones and helps them discover their culinary abilities. It is a stupendous first dish for

noontime or a rich dinner for the summer. With some of your help and a little ability on your part, the stuffed tomatoes will come to be one of their favorite recipes.

- **Age:** 6–12 years
- **Number of participants:** at least one
- **Space:** kitchen
- **Materials:**
  - * 4 medium tomatoes
  - * 4 eggs
  - * bread crumbs
  - * butter
  - * salt
  - * pepper
- **Method:** Ask your child to, after putting on an apron and washing his/her hands, wash the tomatoes under the cold-water faucet.
  Afterward, and with the help of a knife, he/she should cut the upper
  part of the tomatoes, as if he/she were taking off their lids.

  Next he/she can use a dessert spoon to empty the contents of
  the tomatoes to be able to fill them. He/she should sprinkle them
  with a little salt and pepper and, with your help, crack the eggs and
  put one in each tomato. Add a little salt and cover them with bread
  crumbs and a little butter.

  When the tomatoes are filled, distribute them on an oven tray
  or a pan and put them in the oven for about ten minutes, so they
  are at an elevated temperature. When you see that the egg whites
  are cooked, the eggs will be ready to be served as a delicious and
  nutritious first course.

Chicken pie

The oven is a very practical option that allows the kids to cook, but the cooking
point should be monitored and you can help make and take out the dish.

With a little collaboration, your child will be able to make a stupendous dinner and initiate himself/herself into the passionate world of cooking.

- **Age:** 6–12 years
- **Number of participants:** at least one
- **Space:** kitchen
- **Materials:**
  * 2 pounds (1 kg) of chicken fillets, cut very finely
  * very fine bacon slices
  * sliced cheese
  * grated cheese
  * oregano
  * salt
  * dish that goes in the oven
- **Method:** Ask your child to salt the fillets with the help of a saltshaker so that the salt is not in excess. Afterward, he/she should sprinkle them with oregano. With those fillets he/she should cover the bottom of the oven dish. This will be the first layer of the pie. Next, he/she should cover it with slices of bacon and, afterward, with slices of cheese, and then continue once again with the chicken fillets. In all, he/she should put three layers of fillets and it is advisable to have the top layer as bacon. On top of it, he/she should sprinkle grated cheese and put it in the oven at maximum heat for ten minutes. Afterward, you should turn on the grill and cook it au gratin for a couple of minutes, but with your help, the child won't burn himself/herself.

Stuffed eggs

Hard-boiled eggs are usually a food that kids love. They are easy to prepare, they are fun to peel, and their flavor is very smooth. In addition, this is the healthiest way of making them. If you make them stuffed, you increase their nutritional value and you provide your child with an ideal occasion to help you in the kitchen.

- **Age:** 8–12 years
- **Number of participants:** at least one
- **Space:** kitchen
- **Materials:**
    * 4 eggs
    * tuna
    * mayonnaise
    * pickles
    * lettuce
    * knife
    * pot
    * dish
- **Method:** Ask your child to wash the eggs carefully under the faucet. Next, he/she should submerge them in a pot and you should let them boil for ten minutes, until they are converted to hard-boiled eggs that will be the basis of this recipe.

    When the cooked eggs are tepid, tell your child to peel them. Afterward, once you have wet the blade of a knife in water, your child should cut them longitudinally in two halves. He/she should put the yolks on a plate and save the egg whites to start to fill them.

    To make the filling you don't have to use all the yolks, because they would make too much filling upon adding the rest of the ingredients. Once some are set aside, he/she should add the tuna and a little mayonnaise. With the help of a fork, bind the mixture until you have obtained a creamy paste. Afterward, fill the egg whites with this paste until you have formed a little crest. Over each half-stuffed egg put a slice of pickle to adorn and prepare them all in a dish over a finely chopped lettuce base.

Lentil croquettes

Lentils are a rich source of iron, but kids usually don't enjoy them much. Without a doubt, if you propose to your child to eat them in croquettes, and, in addition, that he/she cooks them, it is possible that he/she will eat them happily. You don't lose anything trying it.

- **Age:** 8–12 years
- **Number of participants:** at least one
- **Space:** kitchen
- **Materials:**
    * 1 ¼ cups (250 g) of cooked lentils
    * 1 clove of garlic, chopped
    * 1 spoonful of chopped parsley
    * 1 spoonful of oregano
    * bread crumbs
    * 2 eggs
- **Method:** Your child should place the cooked lentils in a deep dish and crush them with the help of a fork. Afterward, he/she mixes them with the chopped garlic clove, the parsley, and the oregano; then add salt and a little dash of pepper.

    Next, add the necessary bread crumbs to obtain a consistent mixture that your child can mold. With a little skill, he/she can shape the croquettes, with only their hands and two spoons. Afterward, he/she should beat the eggs on a plate and put the bread crumbs on another plate. First put the croquettes into the beaten egg and afterward into the breadcrumbs. Now it is your turn to fry them in abundant hot olive oil. After frying them, put them over absorbent paper to eliminate the excess olive oil, and you can serve them accompanied by a mixed salad.

Wheat gluten (seitan) sandwiches

Although preparing a sandwich seems like a child's thing, the truth is that the sandwich that we propose to you seems like the work of all chefs. In addition, it is a fun way of introducing into their diet very healthy and nutritious foods like seitan. Your child will love the whole process and enjoy the final result, which can be an appetizing dinner.

- **Age:** 9–12 years
- **Number of participants:** at least one
- **Space:** kitchen
- **Materials:**
  * bread
  * butter
  * lettuce
  * tomato for salad
  * slices of cheese
  * seitan
  * mayonnaise
  * olive oil
  * toothpicks
  * toaster
  * knife
  * cutting board
  * frying pan
- **Method:** Ask your child to put the bread in the toaster to brown it a little. Next, he/she should spread a little butter on the bread and put on a slice of cheese. With the help of a knife he/she should cut the lettuce thinly and the tomato into slices. At the base of the sandwich will be a layer of lettuce and a slice of tomato.

Help him/her sauté a little bit of seitan cut into small pieces. Afterward, he/she should shred the seitan with a fork and mix it with a little mayonnaise.

Next, spread it over the slice of tomato, and, finally, put it on the other slice of toasted bread.

When the sandwich is made, he/she should put in a toothpick close to each corner of the slice so that it doesn't dismantle, and cut it into four pieces with the toothpick in the middle of each one of them. Afterward, put them in a dish and you have a healthy, delicious seitan sandwich.

Salmon skewers

As you already know, nutrition is fundamental to kids' development, physically and mentally. Fish plays a very important role in the diet of young people, as it is a very nutritious food, low in calories, and healthy for you. With this simple and delicious recipe you will also create something that your child likes.

- **Age:** 10–12 years
- **Number of participants:** at least one
- **Space:** kitchen
- **Materials:**
    * diced salmon without bones
    * mushrooms
    * green pepper
    * cherry tomatoes
    * dill
    * salt
    * olive oil
    * brochettes
    * knife

* cutting board
* frying pan
- **Method:** Ask at the fish store if they can make you some salmon fillets without bones from the tail. Next, tell your child to cut the fillets into wedges. Afterward, he/she should wash the mushrooms, cherry tomatoes, and green pepper.

  After cutting the green pepper into squares the size of the wedges of salmon, he/she should skewer onto each brochette all the alternating ingredients. Next, help him/her to salt them and to sprinkle them with dill. Afterward, your child can sprinkle them with olive oil.

  Put a frying pan on the stove and put the brochettes on the griddle for one minute on each side. You can present them with a garnish of salted vegetables or a green salad.

Apple pie with a twist

This is a simple pie with a rich flavor and high nutritional content, as it is made with banana, apples, and milk. It can be an ideal dessert, but also a breakfast or snack for your child. To prepare it would be almost as enjoyable as eating it.

- **Age:** 10–12 years
- **Number of participants:** at least one
- **Space:** kitchen
- **Materials:**
    * 4 red apples
    * 2 bananas
    * ½ cup of milk
    * 2 spoonfuls of sugar
    * whipped cream
    * knife
    * cutting board

> * pastry shell
> * electric beater

- **Method:** Ask your child to peel and cut the four apples, into layers. Next, he/she should cover the bottom of the pastry shell completely with the layers of apple and put it in the preheated oven at 425°F (218°C) for about three minutes.

  In the meantime, peel the bananas and cut them into small pieces. Put them in a bowl, add the half cup of milk and the two spoonfuls of sugar, and beat them with the electric beater. The final texture should seem like that of mayonnaise, such that you add more milk if it is too thick. The child should pour the mixture on top of the layers of apple that he/she has cooked previously and let it cool at room temperature if it is winter or for an hour in the refrigerator if it is summer.

Chocolate sponge cake

This is an irresistible recipe that your child will want to make each week. In addition to being a snack or a luxurious breakfast, it can also be a splendid birthday cake with toppings of cream, cherries, and the corresponding candles.

- **Age:** 8–12 years
- **Number of participants:** at least one
- **Space:** kitchen
- **Materials:**
  > * 2 eggs
  > * ⅔ cup (125 g) of brown sugar
  > * 1 cup (150 g) of flour
  > * 1 teaspoon of baking powder
  > * ½ cup (125 g) of olive oil
  > * whipped cream

* cherries
* 2 teaspoons of cocoa powder
* butter
* an 8-inch (20 cm) baking tin

- **Method:** Ask your child to break the two eggs into a wide bowl. Next, he/she should add the cocoa powder and brown sugar, and beat the mixture until he/she has obtained a creamy texture. When he/she has that, pour in the sifted flour and the teaspoon of baking powder, and afterward the olive oil. Ideally, you can beat this final mixture with an electric beater so that it's less taxing on your hands. If you have one at home, help your child use it to ease the work.

  After making the dough, he/she should grease an 8-inch (20 cm) baking tin with butter. When this is well spread, he/she should pour the dough in it and put the baking tin in the preheated oven at 350°F (180°C) for an hour. Ask him/her to poke it with a sharp object or a knife with a small blade to see if the cake is well cooked. The sharp object should be completely clean—if it has residue you should put the cake back in the oven for a little longer.

  Afterward, help him/her take out the cake from the oven and wait for it to cool. Finally, remove it from the mold and decorate it with whipped cream and cherries. Delicious!

Lemon mousse

The kitchen offers many possibilities to develop the creative aptitudes of our little chefs. It requires only your supervision and your desire to put on the apron. Amongst all the recipes, desserts are the most fun when it comes time to put your child in front of the stove. This lemon mousse, in addition, does not require starting the stove, so the participation of your child in this recipe is complete. You will be able to enjoy his/her own creation, and he/she will be very happy to see how you enjoy it with him/her.

- **Age:** 6–12 years
- **Number of participants:** at least one
- **Space:** kitchen
- **Materials:**
    * 3 eggs
    * 1 lemon
    * 1 cup (200 g) of fresh cheese
    * ½ cup (100 g) of brown sugar
    * 4 medium apricots
    * 1 lime
    * beater
    * juicer
    * 2 bowls
    * containers for the mousse
- **Method:** After dividing the eggs in half, help your child pass the yolk from one side to the other to separate it from the egg whites. There is also a small cooking utensil that can help with this.

    Once the whites are separate from the yolks, ask that he/she put them in a bowl and mix them with the fresh cheese, lemon, and brown sugar. To squeeze out the lemon juice, he/she can do it in a manual juicer or in a beater, although he/she can squeeze between his/her hands the two halves with force.

    With the help of a beater, he/she should mix the egg whites, which were separated at the beginning of the recipe, in another bowl until they look like snow. Afterward, mix them with the lemon mixture he/she made before and pour this mixture into the containers, which can be wine glasses or jelly molds. After peeling the apricots, he/she should put each half in each glass to decorate the mousse. He/she can also put on top, if he/she prefers, a slice of lime.

Cookies

With a little of your help, your child can cook some very creative, delicious cookies that his/her friends will love when he/she invites them for a snack. It is a simple recipe that allows them to get to know the kitchen better and enjoy the creation of a dessert that can accompany their breakfasts.

- **Age:** 5–12 years
- **Number of participants:** at least one
- **Space:** kitchen
- **Materials:**
  * ½ cup (120 g) of melted butter
  * powdered sugar
  * 1 egg
  * 1 ½ cups (200 g) of flour
  * to decorate: raisins, grated chocolate, colored sprinkles, almonds . . .
  * a bowl
  * a rolling pin
- **Method:** After covering him/her well with an apron and asking your child to wash his/her hands, teach him/her how to turn on the oven. It should be at 350°F (180°C) during the time that you spend making these sweet and fun cookies.

  Next, ask him/her to mix in a bowl the melted butter, the egg, and the powdered sugar. If you don't find powdered sugar in the store, you can turn regular sugar into powder with the help of a coffee grinder. Without ceasing the mixing, ask your child to add the flour. Once the dough is made, put it on top of the marble, and with the help of a rolling pin or a bottle, he/she should spread it out until it becomes a very thin layer.

And now he/she can start to cut out cookies with the molds, or with a knife. On top, he/she can put on the ingredients that he/she likes to use for decoration. They can be colored sprinkles, powdered sugar, grated chocolate, raisins, almonds, etc.

At the same time that he/she is cutting them he/she should be putting them on the baking sheet that you will have previously coated with flour. Afterward, put the sheet in the oven for half an hour and enjoy a delicious snack.

Fruit with chocolate

Fruit and chocolate skewers are very easy to prepare and make a very original and attractive dessert. They can also constitute a sweet snack for your kids, who will eat the beloved fruits thanks to the taste of the chocolate. It is all a simple and surprising experience to spend a short time in the kitchen together with your kids.

- **Age:** 4–10 years
- **Number of participants:** at least one
- **Space:** kitchen
- **Materials:**
    * 4 chocolate bars a la taza (Spanish hot chocolate)
    * strawberries, grapes, bananas, pears, mandarins . . .
    * lemon juice
    * brochettes
    * a pot
    * a cutting board
- **Method:** Fruit with chocolate is an authentic delight, in addition to an exceptional dessert or snack. And best of all is that your little ones can prepare it almost alone, except for, of course, the melting of the chocolate.

    The preparation is very simple. He/she should put on an apron and wash his/her hands before (excuse the repetition) putting his/her hands to work. This recipe can be made with whatever fruit they like (for example, strawberries, grapes, or mandarin orange pieces in the case of small fruits). Or cut up bigger fruits, like bananas, pears, oranges, or apples. Once ready, they are skewered on the sticks. This can be done with just one fruit or various combinations, playing with colors and textures. Once skewered, they are sprayed with freshly squeezed lemon juice so that they don't go brown.

While they do the initial preparation, you can break apart the chocolate. For that, cut the chocolate into small pieces and place it in a pot. Put in water to boil in a bigger pot and melt the chocolate "bain marie." When it is melted well, tell the kids to wet the brochettes only on a side and let them dry supported by the side that they have not spread with chocolate. And that is it!

Science experiments

Phases of the moon

When kids start to ask why the shape of the moon changes, that is the ideal moment to dedicate time to doing this experiment and discovering the phases of the moon and their relationship with the sun and our planet. With some simple materials and a little imagination, they will be able to get an idea of their place inside our magnificent solar system.

- **Age:** 6–12 years
- **Number of participants:** at least one
- **Space:** a dark room
- **Materials:**
    * a flashlight
    * a tennis ball
    * a cord about 8 inches (20 cm) in length
    * tape
- **Method:** Ask your child to paste the cord to the ball with the help of a little tape. Afterward, tell him/her to sit in the middle of the room and raise the hanging ball from the cord at the height of his/her head. Turn out the light and turn on the flashlight. With the flashlight, illuminate the ball while your child spins it slowly above himself/herself.

And thus the phases of the moon are reproduced. In this experiment, the ball represents the moon, the flashlight is the sun, and the child's head is the earth. The sun always illuminates half the moon and the moon travels around the earth once each month. When the moon is between the earth and the sun, we can't see any reflection of light, which we call a new moon. When the earth is between the sun and the moon, the whole moon can be seen; this is called a full moon.

With this experiment, you will have spent a good time and it will surely help your child study the phases of the moon when he/she explains it in school.

Magic balloon

Many substances exist in the home that, mixed, produce completely unexpected effects. When you show your child what bicarbonate mixed with vinegar is capable of doing, he/she will think that a magic trick has been accomplished, but in reality it is, simply, a chemical reaction with a surprising result. Surely it will become a favorite trick for family table talk.

- **Age:** 4–10 years
- **Number of participants:** at least one
- **Space:** wherever
- **Materials:**
  * a balloon
  * a clear, crystal, medium-sized jar with a little bit of a neck
  * 4 teaspoons of bicarbonate
  * vinegar
  * a teaspoon
- **Method:** Tell your child to fill the jar halfway with vinegar. Next, he/she can add the four teaspoons of bicarbonate inside the balloon

with the help of a funnel. Afterward, he/she should put the mouth of the balloon on the neck of the jar using tape, but avoid at all cost letting a single speck of bicarbonate inside of the jar.

Once the balloon is fixed well on the neck of the jar, help your child raise the balloon in a way that all the bicarbonate contained in the balloon drops into the vinegar. When both substances are mixed, the vinegar starts to bubble and the gas that the chemical reaction gives off starts to swell the balloon. Carbon dioxide is responsible for the process, and it can result in higher or lower amounts depending on how much bicarbonate you add.

Create a rainbow

Since kids were very little, rainbows fascinated them. It is one of the great diversions on those rare occasions in which sunlight and rain are combined. Surely a boring afternoon can be full of color if you propose to your child to create his/her own rainbow and express it in a splendid work of art. There is no doubt that it will be a trick that, later, your little one will use to impress his/her friends.

- **Age:** 3–10 years
- **Number of participants:** at least one
- **Space:** wherever
- **Materials:**
    * a long, straight, transparent glass cup
    * a white piece of paper
    * water
    * colored pencils
    * flashlight
- **Method:** This magic trick, which we are calling a physics experiment about the refraction of light, can be made using natural sunlight or a flashlight.

Firstly, the child should fill the cup with water a bit more than halfway. If you decide to do the experiment on a day without sunlight, you should look for a room in the house that can stay completely dark and use a flashlight.

Next, lean the white sheet on a wall, or hold it up yourself, and place the cup of water at a distance of about 8 inches (20 cm). With the lit flashlight, ask your child to project the light on the paper but through the cup, so that the light goes through the water in the glass. As a result of the decomposition of the light in the prism that the water makes, he/she will see the rainbow reflected on the paper. If it is not visible at first, move the sheet a bit until the colors materialize on it.

Afterward, you can ask your child to draw the rainbow that he/she has created on another sheet, as a memory of this fun and simple science experiment.

> **Variable:** If you decide to do it on a sunny afternoon, you should choose a sunny window so the rays cross the glass of water and are broken down into the rainbow on the paper.

Water cycle

Although this activity requires a little bit of patience, it can be done in two phases and allows time to pass more quickly. You can initiate the experiment before having a snack and test the results after having your cookies, or do it before and after a bath. In whichever case, the result is worth the pain since, in addition to being entertained, your child will learn firsthand one of the most common, but invisible, processes of nature. Included is a good way to teach them the concepts of condensation and evaporation.

- **Age:** 7–10 years

- **Number of participants:** at least one
- **Space:** wherever
- **Materials:**
  - a crystal jar with a medium-sized, clear cover
  - a small plant
  - a lid of a plastic bottle or small glass
  - dirt
  - sand
  - small rocks
- **Method:** Help your child put a layer of small rocks on the bottom of the jar. Next, he/she has to put a fine layer of sand, and afterward he/she should add another layer of dirt. You should be sure that the three layers cover less than half of the jar to guarantee the success of the experiment.

  Once the three layers are prepared, he/she should put the little plant on top and, at its side, the bottle lid or the small glass full of water. All prepared now, your child should cover the jar well and put it in the sun.

  The sun will make the water evaporate and empty the glass. That evaporated water will condense on the cover of the jar until forming small drops, which will fall like rain above the plant when its weight obliges them or they will trickle down the walls of the jar and will wet the rocks, sand, and dirt, providing the water that the plant needs through its roots. You will have created a mini biosphere and you will be able to contemplate the water cycle from start to finish.

Create a tornado

Nature is prodigious and encompasses many mysteries yet to be resolved. Without a doubt, others are known and, although they seem like magic, your child can reproduce them in his/her own house. An example is the tornado. With the experiment that we propose to you next, you can teach your child to create it and understand the forces that act in this meteorological phenomenon.

- **Age:** 9–12 years
- **Number of participants:** at least one
- **Space:** wherever
- **Materials:**
  * big plastic bottle of soda with its cap
  * water
  * olive oil
  * black pepper
  * bowl
  * spoon
  * funnel
  * stamp/something to puncture the cap
  * paper and pencil
- **Method:** The child should mix the water with a little olive oil in the bowl. Afterward, tell him/her to add a little pepper.

  Next, fill a little more than half the plastic bottle with water and add a little bit of the mixture until leaving only a quarter of the bottle free. He/she can help with a funnel if necessary.

  After filling it, he/she should make a hole ⅕–¼ inch (5–6 mm) in diameter in the bottle cap, place it on the bottle, and close it well.

  To finish the experiment, he/she should cover the hole with his/her finger at the top so that the water doesn't fall and turn the bottle over. Next, he/she should turn it over himself/herself many times.

  Keeping the bottle mouth down, he/she should raise his/her finger from the lid and let the water fall. The olive oil will form a whirlpool, or vortex, and it will drag the particles of pepper that it finds in its path. Your child will have just created a tornado in the bottle.

Conserve a drop of rain

This surprising experiment permits your child to do something as incredible as saving raindrops. It is a magnificent excuse to convert a tiresome rainy afternoon to a scientific discovery.

- **Age:** 9–12 years
- **Number of participants:** at least one
- **Space:** at home, on a rainy afternoon
- **Materials:**
  - * flour
  - * frying pan
  - * rainwater
  - * skimmer
  - * power source for the oven
- **Method:** The first thing you need is, evidently, for it to be raining. If this happens, ask your child to cover the bottom of a frying pan with flour to a height of about ⁸⁄₁₀ inch (2 cm). He/she will love this phase, because all little ones like to play with flour, but the following is going to fascinate them.

    Next, turn on the oven to the maximum temperature so it gets hot. Open a window, or go on the terrace, with the frying pan so the child can expose it to the rain and allow the drops to fall inside the floured surface. When he/she has them, return to the kitchen, and with the help of a skimmer or a spoon with holes, ask him/her to "gather" the small balls of flour that the raindrops have created. These drops should be put inside the oven. The temperature will make them harden in just a few minutes and, when they are fried, the child will learn what form the raindrops have when they fall to the ground, and their new texture will permit him/her to conserve them and show them to his/her friends.

Create your own telephone

The telephone is one of the most utilized objects these days, especially cell phones. With this experiment, your child will be able to create his/her own project that is similar to what we had made as little ones, and communicate with you or with his/her friends through the art of magic.

- **Age:** 6–12 years
- **Number of participants:** at least two
- **Space:** wherever
- **Materials:**
    * 2 plastic yogurt cups
    * paper
    * colored pencils
    * a piece of rope or yarn
    * glue
- **Method:** Wrap the yogurt cups with a piece of paper that the children have previously decorated. It can be a free drawing or coloring of a motif that you yourself propose. Afterward, with the help of a burin or some sharp scissors, make a hole in the center of the base of the plastic cups. In those holes the kids should tie the piece of rope or yarn of approximately 3 ⅓ feet (1 m). And thus all the material that composes the telephone has been built. Now the kids will be able to communicate amongst themselves or with you. How? Well, while one child talks through a cup, the other will listen through the second cup. Thus, it is simple.

Floating egg

Science experiments can be very complicated, or as simple as this one. With it you will be able to teach your child that objects float with ease in salty water, but sink in regular water. Simple and effective.

- **Age:** 8–12 years
- **Number of participants:** at least one
- **Space:** wherever
- **Materials:**
    * an egg
    * a glass
    * water
    * salt
    * a spoon
- **Method:** Put very salty water halfway up the glass, and, cautiously, regular water, so that the two don't mix. Next, tell your child to deposit, cautiously, the egg inside of the glass and he/she will be able to test if it will float between the two waters. If you add a little more salt to the bottom of the glass with a straw, then the egg will float upward. On the other hand, if what you poured is regular water on the surface, the egg will sink. With that you will be able to demonstrate to your child why it is easier to float in ocean water than in the pool.

Making cheese

It is probable that your child asks at some point how cheese, which is solid, is made, since milk is of a liquid consistency. With this experiment you will be able to imitate the process that the farmers have used to make cheese and your child will understand how he/she can convert milk to cheese.

- **Age:** 8–12 years
- **Number of participants:** at least one
- **Space:** kitchen
- **Materials:**
    * 2 cups (½ l) of milk
    * 1 tablespoon of vinegar

* coffee filter
* 1 crystal jar with a cover
* 1 small container

- **Method:** First you should pour a cup of milk into the crystal jar. Next add to it a tablespoon of vinegar and close the jar well with the lid. Ask your child to shake it forcefully so that it is all mixed well. It will become a lumpy mixture in which the milk has transformed into liquid and lumps.

  Place the coffee filter in the other container and submerge it with your hand so that the filter doesn't fall inside while you do the next step. Now, cautiously pour the mixture into the filter. He/she should do it slowly, realizing that he/she has to pour a part of the mixture, wait for it to filter, and afterward add the rest.

  Once the filtering is done, join the two sides of the filter cautiously and squeeze out the rest of the liquid. Lumps should stay in the filter. Squeeze them and . . . now you have cheese! But don't eat it—it is only an experiment.

Balancing forks

This experiment requires a little skill, but the result looks like the work of a magician and your child will like to teach it to his/her friends. With the help of the water he/she will be able to maintain in balance something as heavy as two metal forks, without anyone's help.

- **Age:** 10–12 years
- **Number of participants:** at least one
- **Space:** wherever
- **Materials:**
    * 2 metal forks
    * clay or Play-Doh
    * flat toothpick

           * wide-mouthed cup

           * water

- **Method:** First your child should make a ball of clay or Play-Doh the size of a big, firmly compacted marble. Afterward, tell him/her to introduce the point of one of the forks into the ball of clay, and, next, the other fork, forming a forty-five-degree angle, into the first. Afterward, he/she should stick the flat toothpick under the clay ball situated between the forks. With this, the device that will be put in equilibrium to the forks is equipped.

  Now, he/she should place the other side of the toothpick in the base of the cup and move it around the base of the cup until obtaining the equilibrium of the forks. If the forks are not balanced, he/she should reduce the angle between them and make the necessary adjustments until they are balanced.

  Explain to him/her that the reason that the balance of the two forks is obtained is, precisely, a result of the angle that has been created between them, since all the weight is concentrated in the toothpick and is kept upright. The reason this happens is the center of gravity of the ensemble.